The Power Hustle: a Guide to Balancing Work and Fitness for Women

The Power of Exercise

1.1 Understanding the Benefits of Exercise

Exercise is not just about losing weight or achieving a certain body shape. It is a powerful tool that can positively impact every aspect of a woman's life, especially when it comes to balancing work and fitness. In this section, we will explore the numerous benefits of exercise and how it can enhance your physical, mental, and emotional well-being.

Physical Benefits

Regular exercise offers a wide range of physical benefits that can improve your overall health and well-being. Here are some of the key advantages:

1. **Increased Energy Levels**: Engaging in physical activity boosts your energy levels by improving blood circulation and oxygen flow throughout your body. This increased energy can help you stay focused and productive throughout your workday.

2. **Improved Strength and Endurance**: Exercise helps build muscle strength and endurance, making everyday tasks easier to accomplish. Whether it's carrying groceries, lifting heavy objects, or simply staying active throughout the day, being physically strong and fit can greatly enhance your work performance.

3. **Enhanced Cardiovascular Health**: Regular cardiovascular exercise, such as running, swimming, or cycling, strengthens your heart and improves its efficiency. This reduces the risk of heart disease, lowers blood pressure, and increases your overall cardiovascular fitness.

4. **Weight Management**: Exercise plays a crucial role in maintaining a healthy weight. By burning calories and increasing your metabolic rate, regular physical activity can help you achieve and maintain a healthy body weight, which is essential for overall well-being.

5. **Improved Sleep Quality**: Engaging in regular exercise can improve the quality of your sleep. Physical activity helps regulate your sleep patterns, making it easier for you to fall asleep and stay asleep throughout the night. This, in turn, can enhance your productivity and focus during the day.

Mental and Emotional Benefits

Exercise not only benefits your physical health but also has a profound impact on your mental and emotional well-being. Here are some of the ways exercise can positively affect your mind:

1. **Reduced Stress and Anxiety**: Exercise is a natural stress reliever. It stimulates the production of endorphins, also known as "feel-good" hormones, which help reduce stress and anxiety levels. Regular physical activity can provide a much-needed break from work-related stress and help you maintain a positive mindset.

2. **Improved Mood and Mental Clarity**: Exercise has been shown to boost mood and improve mental clarity. It increases the production of neurotransmitters like serotonin and dopamine, which are responsible for regulating mood and promoting feelings of happiness and well-being. This can have a significant impact on your work performance and overall satisfaction.

3. **Enhanced Cognitive Function**: Regular exercise has been linked to improved cognitive function, including enhanced memory, focus, and concentration. Engaging in physical activity increases blood flow to the brain, promoting the growth of new brain cells and improving overall brain health.

4. **Increased Self-Confidence**: Regular exercise can boost your self-confidence and self-esteem. As you achieve your fitness goals and witness improvements in your physical abilities, you develop a sense of accomplishment and pride. This newfound confidence can positively impact your work life, allowing you to take on challenges with a greater sense of self-assurance.

5. **Stress Relief and Relaxation**: Exercise provides an opportunity to disconnect from work-related stressors and focus on yourself. Whether it's going for a run, practicing yoga, or engaging in any form of physical activity, exercise can serve as a form of relaxation and stress relief. It allows you to clear your mind, recharge, and return to work with a renewed sense of energy and focus.

Long-Term Health Benefits

In addition to the immediate physical, mental, and emotional benefits, regular exercise also offers long-term health advantages. By incorporating exercise into your daily routine, you can reduce the risk of various chronic diseases and improve your overall quality of life. Some of the long-term health benefits of exercise include:

1. **Reduced Risk of Chronic Diseases**: Regular physical activity can lower the risk of developing chronic conditions such as heart disease, type 2 diabetes, certain types of cancer, and osteoporosis. Exercise helps maintain healthy blood pressure, cholesterol levels, and blood sugar levels, reducing the risk of these diseases.

2. **Improved Bone Health**: Weight-bearing exercises, such as walking, jogging, and strength training, help strengthen bones and reduce the risk of osteoporosis. As women age, maintaining strong bones becomes increasingly important, and exercise plays a crucial role in achieving this.

3. **Enhanced Immune Function**: Regular exercise can boost your immune system, making you less susceptible to common illnesses and infections. Physical activity increases the production of antibodies and white blood cells, which help fight off bacteria and viruses.

4. **Reduced Risk of Cognitive Decline**: Engaging in regular exercise has been shown to reduce the risk of cognitive decline and improve brain health as you age. It can help prevent conditions such as Alzheimer's disease and dementia, keeping your mind sharp and functioning optimally.

5. **Increased Longevity**: Leading an active lifestyle has been associated with increased longevity. Regular exercise, combined with a healthy diet and lifestyle, can significantly improve your chances of living a longer, healthier life.

Understanding the benefits of exercise is the first step towards incorporating it into your busy work-life schedule. By prioritizing your physical and mental well-being, you can achieve a better work-life balance and experience the transformative power of exercise. In the following sections, we will explore strategies to find motivation, set realistic fitness goals, and create an exercise routine that fits seamlessly into your busy life.

1.2 Finding Motivation to Exercise

Motivation is the driving force behind any successful endeavor, and when it comes to exercise, finding the motivation to get started and stay consistent can be a challenge, especially for busy working women. However, with the right mindset and strategies, you can tap into your inner motivation and make exercise a regular part of your life. In this section, we will explore various techniques to help you find the motivation you need to prioritize fitness and make it a sustainable habit.

Understanding the Benefits of Exercise

Before we dive into finding motivation, it's important to understand the numerous benefits that exercise can bring to your life. Regular physical activity not only improves your physical health but also has a positive impact on your mental and emotional well-being. Exercise helps to:

1. Boost energy levels: Engaging in physical activity increases blood flow and oxygen delivery to your muscles, which can leave you feeling more energized throughout the day.

2. Reduce stress and anxiety: Exercise releases endorphins, which are natural mood boosters. It can help alleviate stress and anxiety, promoting a sense of calm and relaxation.

3. Improve mental clarity and focus: Physical activity stimulates brain function, enhancing cognitive abilities such as memory, attention, and problem-solving skills.

4. Enhance self-confidence: Regular exercise can improve body image and self-esteem, helping you feel more confident and comfortable in your own skin.

5. Increase productivity: When you exercise regularly, you'll notice an improvement in your ability to concentrate and be more productive at work.

6. Promote better sleep: Physical activity can help regulate your sleep patterns, leading to more restful and rejuvenating sleep.

7. Strengthen the immune system: Regular exercise boosts the immune system, reducing the risk of illness and improving overall health.

8. Maintain a healthy weight: Exercise, combined with a balanced diet, can help you achieve and maintain a healthy weight, reducing the risk of chronic diseases such as heart disease and diabetes.

Finding Your Inner Motivation

Motivation is deeply personal, and what inspires one person may not work for another. It's essential to identify your own reasons for wanting to exercise and tap into your inner motivation. Here are some strategies to help you find your drive:

1. Set meaningful goals: Define what you want to achieve through exercise. Whether it's improving your overall fitness, losing weight, or training for a specific event, having clear goals will give you something to work towards and keep you motivated.

2. Find activities you enjoy: Experiment with different types of exercise until you find activities that you genuinely enjoy. When you

look forward to your workouts, it becomes easier to stay motivated
and make exercise a regular part of your routine.

3. Create a positive mindset: Cultivate a positive attitude towards
exercise by focusing on the benefits it brings to your life. Instead of
viewing it as a chore, reframe it as an opportunity to take care of
yourself and invest in your well-being.

4. Surround yourself with support: Seek out like-minded individuals
who share your fitness goals or join a fitness community. Surrounding
yourself with supportive people can provide encouragement, accountability, and motivation on your fitness journey.

5. Track your progress: Keep a record of your workouts, noting your
achievements and improvements along the way. Seeing your progress
can be incredibly motivating and help you stay committed to your
fitness routine.

6. Reward yourself: Set up a system of rewards for reaching milestones
or sticking to your exercise routine. Treat yourself to something you
enjoy, like a massage, a new workout outfit, or a relaxing day off.

7. Visualize success: Take a few moments each day to visualize yourself
achieving your fitness goals. Imagine how you will feel, the sense of
accomplishment, and the positive impact it will have on your life.
Visualization can be a powerful tool for motivation.

8. Make it a habit: Consistency is key when it comes to exercise.
Make it a non-negotiable part of your daily or weekly routine. By
establishing a habit, it becomes easier to stay motivated as it becomes
second nature.

Overcoming Obstacles and Excuses

Even with the best intentions, obstacles and excuses can get in the way of
your exercise routine. It's important to anticipate and address these challenges
head-on. Here are some common obstacles and strategies to overcome them:

Lack of time: Time is often cited as the biggest barrier to exercise.
However, with proper time management and prioritization, you can
carve out time for physical activity. Consider waking up earlier,
utilizing your lunch break, or finding pockets of time throughout the
day to fit in short workouts.

Fatigue: Long work hours and demanding schedules can leave you feeling exhausted. However, exercise can actually boost your energy levels. Start with shorter, less intense workouts and gradually increase the duration and intensity as your energy levels improve.

Lack of motivation: There will be days when you simply don't feel like exercising. On those days, remind yourself of your goals, the benefits of exercise, and how good you'll feel afterward. Sometimes, taking that first step is all it takes to get motivated.

Weather conditions: Inclement weather can make it challenging to exercise outdoors. Have a backup plan for indoor workouts, such as home workout videos, online classes, or investing in exercise equipment like a treadmill or stationary bike.

Work-related stress: High levels of stress can make it difficult to find the motivation to exercise. However, exercise is an excellent stress reliever. Consider incorporating stress-reducing activities like yoga or meditation into your routine to help manage work-related stress. Remember, motivation may ebb and flow, but by understanding the benefits of exercise, finding your inner drive, and overcoming obstacles, you can stay motivated and make exercise a consistent part of your life.

1.3 Setting Realistic Fitness Goals

Setting realistic fitness goals is an essential step in achieving success on your fitness journey. Without clear goals, it can be challenging to stay motivated and focused. In this section, we will explore the importance of setting realistic fitness goals and provide you with practical tips to help you set goals that are achievable and sustainable.

Why Set Fitness Goals?

Setting fitness goals provides you with a clear direction and purpose for your workouts. It helps you stay motivated, track your progress, and celebrate your achievements along the way. Here are a few reasons why setting fitness goals is crucial:

1. **Motivation:** Goals give you something to strive for and keep you motivated during challenging times. When you have a specific goal in mind, it becomes easier to push through obstacles and stay committed to your fitness routine.

2. **Focus:** Setting goals helps you prioritize your efforts and focus on what truly matters. It allows you to structure your workouts and make informed decisions about the types of exercises and activities that will help you reach your desired outcome.

3. **Measurable Progress:** Goals provide a benchmark for measuring your progress. By setting specific targets, you can track your achievements and see how far you've come. This sense of progress can be incredibly motivating and encourage you to keep pushing forward.

4. **Accountability:** When you set goals, you hold yourself accountable for your actions. Having a clear objective makes it easier to stay committed and disciplined, as you have a tangible target to work towards.

Tips for Setting Realistic Fitness Goals

Now that you understand the importance of setting fitness goals, let's explore some practical tips to help you set goals that are realistic and achievable:

1. **Be Specific:** Set clear and specific goals that outline exactly what you want to achieve. For example, instead of saying, "I want to get fit," specify your goal as, "I want to be able to run a 5K race in under 30 minutes."

2. **Make Them Measurable:** Ensure your goals are measurable so that you can track your progress. This could include metrics such as weight loss, body measurements, or the number of repetitions or sets you can perform for a particular exercise.

3. **Set Realistic Timeframes:** Give yourself enough time to achieve your goals without feeling overwhelmed. Setting unrealistic timeframes can lead to frustration and disappointment. Break down your goals into smaller milestones and set a timeline that is both challenging and attainable.

4. **Consider Your Current Fitness Level:** Take into account your current fitness level when setting goals. It's important to be realistic about what you can achieve based on your starting point. Gradually increase the intensity and duration of your workouts as you progress.

5. **Focus on Process Goals:** In addition to outcome goals, set process goals that focus on the actions and behaviors necessary to achieve your desired outcome. For example, instead of solely focusing on losing a certain amount of weight, set a process goal of exercising for 30 minutes five times a week.

6. **Make Goals Personal and Meaningful:** Your goals should align with your personal values and aspirations. When your goals have personal significance, you are more likely to stay committed and motivated to achieve them.

7. **Break Goals into Smaller Steps:** Break down your larger goals into smaller, more manageable steps. This allows you to track your progress more effectively and provides a sense of accomplishment as you achieve each milestone.

8. **Be Flexible and Adjust as Needed:** It's essential to be flexible and

adjust your goals as needed. Life can throw unexpected challenges your way, and it's important to adapt your goals accordingly. Be open to modifying your goals if necessary, while still maintaining a sense of focus and determination.

Remember, setting realistic fitness goals is not about perfection but about progress. Celebrate each milestone you achieve along the way and use setbacks as opportunities to learn and grow. With a clear vision and realistic goals, you can create a fitness routine that is both enjoyable and sustainable.

1.4 Creating an Exercise Routine

Creating an exercise routine is an essential step in achieving your fitness goals and maintaining a healthy lifestyle as a working woman. By establishing a consistent exercise routine, you can ensure that you prioritize your physical well-being and make time for regular physical activity. In this section, we will explore the key elements of creating an effective exercise routine that fits seamlessly into your busy schedule.

Understanding Your Schedule and Commitments

The first step in creating an exercise routine is to assess your schedule and commitments. As a working woman, you likely have various responsibilities and time constraints. Take some time to evaluate your daily and weekly schedule, identifying any windows of time that can be dedicated to exercise. Consider your work hours, family commitments, and other obligations that may impact your availability.

Once you have a clear understanding of your schedule, determine how many days per week you can realistically commit to exercise. Aim for a minimum of three to four days per week to ensure you are getting enough physical activity to reap the benefits. Remember, consistency is key when it comes to exercise, so choose a realistic number of days that you can commit to in the long term.

Setting Realistic Goals

Before diving into creating your exercise routine, it's important to set realistic goals. Think about what you want to achieve through exercise. Do you want to improve your overall fitness, lose weight, build strength, or increase your endurance? Setting specific and achievable goals will help you stay motivated and focused.

Once you have identified your goals, break them down into smaller, manageable milestones. For example, if your goal is to run a 5K race, start by aiming to run for 10 minutes without stopping, then gradually increase your running time each week. By setting smaller goals along the way, you can track your progress and celebrate your achievements, which will keep you motivated to continue with your exercise routine.

Choosing the Right Types of Exercise

When creating your exercise routine, it's important to choose activities that you enjoy and that align with your fitness goals. There are various types of exercise to consider, including cardiovascular exercises (such as running, cycling, or swimming), strength training (using weights or resistance bands), flexibility exercises (such as yoga or Pilates), and high-intensity interval training (HIIT).

Incorporating a combination of these exercises into your routine can provide a well-rounded approach to fitness. For example, you might choose to do cardiovascular exercises three days a week, strength training two days a week, and flexibility exercises one day a week. Experiment with different activities to find what you enjoy and what works best for your body.

Structuring Your Exercise Routine

Now that you have a clear understanding of your schedule, goals, and preferred types of exercise, it's time to structure your exercise routine. Start by determining the duration of each workout session. Aim for at least 30 minutes of moderate-intensity exercise per session, or 150 minutes per week, as recommended by the American Heart Association.

Next, decide on the specific days and times that you will dedicate to exercise. Consider your energy levels throughout the day and choose a time when you are most likely to be consistent and motivated. Some women prefer to exercise in the morning before work, while others find it more convenient to exercise during their lunch break or in the evening. Find what works best for you and stick to that schedule as much as possible.

To ensure variety and prevent boredom, consider incorporating different types of exercise on different days. For example, you might choose to do cardiovascular exercises on Mondays, Wednesdays, and Fridays, strength training on Tuesdays and Thursdays, and flexibility exercises on Saturdays. This way, you can target different muscle groups and keep your workouts interesting.

Staying Accountable and Motivated

Creating an exercise routine is one thing, but sticking to it is another. To stay accountable and motivated, consider implementing strategies that will help you stay on track. One effective strategy is to find an exercise buddy or join a fitness class or group. Exercising with others can provide support, encouragement, and a sense of accountability.

Tracking your progress is another powerful motivator. Keep a workout journal or use a fitness app to record your workouts, track your progress, and celebrate your achievements. Seeing how far you've come can be incredibly motivating and inspire you to keep pushing forward.

Lastly, be flexible and adaptable. Life can sometimes throw unexpected curve-balls, and it's important to be able to adjust your exercise routine when needed. If you miss a workout or have to reschedule, don't beat yourself up. Instead, focus on getting back on track as soon as possible and maintaining a positive mindset.

By creating an exercise routine that fits seamlessly into your busy schedule, you are taking a proactive step towards prioritizing your physical well-being. Remember, consistency is key, so make a commitment to yourself and stick to your routine as much as possible. With time and dedication, you will reap the rewards of a balanced and healthy lifestyle.

Balancing Work and Fitness

2.1 Time Management Strategies

As a busy working woman, finding time to exercise can often feel like an impossible task. Between work responsibilities, family commitments, and personal obligations, it can be challenging to carve out time for yourself and prioritize your fitness goals. However, with effective time management strategies, you can create a schedule that allows you to balance work and fitness without feeling overwhelmed. Here are some tips to help you manage your time effectively and make exercise a non-negotiable part of your routine:

1. Prioritize Your Health and Fitness

The first step in effective time management is to prioritize your health and fitness. Understand that taking care of yourself is not selfish but essential for your overall well-being. Recognize the importance of exercise in maintaining your physical and mental health, and make it a non-negotiable part of your daily routine. By placing a high value on your health, you will be more motivated to find time for exercise.

2. Set Clear Goals and Create a Schedule

To effectively manage your time, it's crucial to set clear fitness goals and create a schedule that aligns with those goals. Start by identifying what you want to achieve through exercise, whether it's improving your strength, losing weight, or increasing your energy levels. Once you have defined your goals, break them down into smaller, actionable steps. Then, create a weekly or monthly schedule that includes dedicated time for exercise. Treat these exercise sessions as important appointments that cannot be missed.

3. Identify Time-Wasting Activities

Take a close look at your daily routine and identify any time-wasting activities that can be eliminated or minimized. This could include excessive time spent on social media, watching TV, or engaging in unproductive conversations. By identifying these time-wasters, you can reclaim valuable minutes or even hours that can be dedicated to exercise. Consider setting limits on your screen time or finding alternative activities that align with your fitness goals.

4. Make the Most of Your Mornings

Mornings can be a great time to fit in a workout before the demands of the day take over. Wake up a little earlier and use this time to engage in physical activity. Whether it's going for a run, practicing yoga, or doing a quick home workout, starting your day with exercise can boost your energy levels and set a positive tone for the rest of the day. Prepare your workout clothes and equipment the night before to make it easier to get started in the morning.

5. Incorporate Exercise into Your Daily Routine

Look for opportunities to incorporate exercise into your daily routine. This could mean taking the stairs instead of the elevator, walking or biking to work, or scheduling walking meetings instead of sitting in a conference room. Find creative ways to move your body throughout the day, even if you have a sedentary job. Set reminders on your phone or use fitness apps to prompt you to take short breaks and engage in physical activity.

6. Delegate and Outsource

Recognize that you don't have to do everything yourself. Delegate tasks at work and at home to free up time for exercise. Whether it's asking a colleague for assistance on a project or hiring help for household chores, delegating responsibilities can give you the time and mental space to focus on your fitness goals. Remember, it's okay to ask for help and prioritize your well-being.

7. Be Flexible and Adapt

Life is unpredictable, and there will be days when your schedule gets disrupted. It's important to be flexible and adapt to these changes without giving up on your fitness goals. If you miss a workout, don't beat yourself up about it. Instead, find alternative ways to stay active, such as taking a brisk walk during your lunch break or doing a quick workout at home. Embrace the concept of progress, not perfection, and remember that consistency is key.

8. Plan and Prepare in Advance

Planning and preparation are essential for effective time management. Take some time each week to plan your workouts and meals in advance. This will help you stay organized and ensure that you have everything you need to make your fitness journey a success. Prepare your gym bag, pack healthy snacks, and plan your meals to avoid last-minute decisions that may derail your progress.

By being proactive, you can eliminate unnecessary stress and make exercise a seamless part of your routine.

9. Practice Self-Care and Rest

While it's important to make time for exercise, it's equally crucial to prioritize self-care and rest. Recognize that rest and recovery are essential components of a balanced fitness routine. Schedule regular rest days to allow your body to recover and prevent burnout. Prioritize sleep and ensure that you are getting enough restorative rest each night. By taking care of your overall well-being, you will have the energy and motivation to stay consistent with your exercise routine.

10. Stay Accountable and Seek Support

Lastly, staying accountable and seeking support can significantly impact your time management and overall success in balancing work and fitness. Find an accountability partner, whether it's a friend, family member, or colleague, who shares similar fitness goals. Share your progress, challenges, and victories with them, and hold each other accountable. Consider joining fitness communities or online groups where you can connect with like-minded individuals who can provide support and motivation.

By implementing these time management strategies, you can effectively balance work and fitness as a busy working woman. Remember, it's not about finding time; it's about making time for what truly matters to you. Prioritize your health, set clear goals, and create a schedule that allows you to incorporate exercise into your daily routine. With dedication, consistency, and a proactive approach, you can achieve a harmonious balance between work and fitness, empowering yourself to live a healthier and more fulfilling life.

2.2 Prioritizing Self-Care

In the hustle and bustle of our daily lives, it's easy for self-care to take a backseat. As a working woman, you may find yourself constantly juggling multiple responsibilities and putting the needs of others before your own. However, it's important to remember that self-care is not selfish; it is essential for your overall well-being and success. Prioritizing self-care is crucial in maintaining a healthy work-life balance and ensuring that you have the energy and resilience to tackle the challenges that come your way.

The Importance of Self-Care

Self-care encompasses a wide range of activities and practices that promote physical, mental, and emotional well-being. It involves taking intentional actions to nurture and care for yourself, both physically and mentally. Many women tend to neglect self-care because they feel guilty or believe that they don't have enough time. However, neglecting self-care can lead to burnout, decreased productivity, and a decline in overall health.

Prioritizing self-care is not only beneficial for your own well-being but also for those around you. When you take care of yourself, you are better equipped to handle stress, make sound decisions, and maintain healthy relationships. By investing time and energy into self-care, you are investing in your own happiness and success.

Creating a Personal Wellness Routine

Prioritizing self-care starts with creating a personal wellness routine that works for you. This routine should include activities and practices that nourish your mind, body, and soul. Here are some key elements to consider when designing your wellness routine:

1. Physical Activity Regular exercise is a vital component of self-care. It not only improves your physical health but also boosts your mood and reduces stress. Find a form of exercise that you enjoy and make it a priority in your routine. Whether it's going for a run, attending a yoga class, or dancing to your favorite music, find an activity that makes you feel good and incorporate it into your schedule.

2. Rest and Relaxation In our fast-paced society, rest and relaxation often take a backseat. However, getting enough sleep and taking time to relax are essential for recharging your body and mind. Prioritize quality sleep by establishing a consistent sleep schedule and creating a relaxing bedtime routine. Additionally, incorporate relaxation techniques such as deep breathing, meditation, or taking a warm bath into your daily routine to help reduce stress and promote relaxation.

3. Healthy Eating Proper nutrition plays a significant role in self-care. Fueling your body with nutritious foods not only supports your physical health but also enhances your mental and emotional well-being. Make an effort to eat a balanced diet that includes a variety of fruits, vegetables, whole grains, lean proteins, and healthy fats. Avoid skipping meals and opt for nourishing snacks to keep your energy levels stable throughout the day.

4. Mindfulness and Stress Reduction Practicing mindfulness and stress reduction techniques can help you stay present, manage stress, and improve your overall well-being. Incorporate activities such as meditation, deep breathing exercises, journaling, or engaging in hobbies that bring you joy into your daily routine. These practices can help you cultivate a sense of calm and clarity amidst the chaos of daily life.

5. Social Connection Nurturing your relationships and fostering social connections is an important aspect of self-care. Make time for meaningful interactions with loved ones, friends, and colleagues. Schedule regular catch-ups, plan outings, or join social groups or clubs that align with your interests. Connecting with others can provide emotional support, boost your mood, and enhance your overall sense of well-being.

6. Personal Time Carving out personal time for yourself is crucial for self-care. This time allows you to engage in activities that bring you joy, recharge your batteries, and pursue your passions. Whether it's reading a book, taking a walk in nature, practicing a hobby, or simply enjoying a cup of tea, make it a priority to set aside dedicated time for yourself each day.

Making Self-Care a Priority

While it may seem challenging to prioritize self-care amidst your busy schedule, it is essential to make it a non-negotiable part of your routine. Here are some strategies to help you make self-care a priority:

1. Set Boundaries Learn to say no and set boundaries to protect your time and energy. It's okay to decline certain commitments or delegate tasks to others. By setting boundaries, you create space for self-care activities and ensure that your needs are met.

2. Schedule Self-Care Treat self-care activities as important appointments and schedule them into your calendar. Block off dedicated time for exercise, relaxation, and personal activities. By treating self-care as a priority, you are more likely to follow through and make it a regular part of your routine.

3. Start Small If you're new to prioritizing self-care, start with small, manageable steps. Begin by incorporating one self-care activity into your routine and gradually build from there. Remember, self-care is a journey, and it's okay to start small and gradually increase your self-care practices over time.

4. Seek Support Don't be afraid to ask for help or seek support from others. Reach out to friends, family, or colleagues who can provide encouragement and accountability. Consider joining a support group or seeking guidance from a coach or therapist who can help you navigate the challenges of balancing work and self-care.

5. Practice Self-Compassion Be kind to yourself and practice self-compassion. Remember that self-care is not selfish; it is necessary for your well-being. Give yourself permission to prioritize your needs and let go of any guilt or self-judgment that may arise.

By prioritizing self-care, you are investing in your own well-being and setting the foundation for a balanced and fulfilling life. Remember, you deserve to take care of yourself, and by doing so, you will be better equipped to handle the demands of work and life with grace and resilience.

2.3 Incorporating Exercise into Your Workday

As a busy working woman, finding time to exercise can often feel like an impossible task. Between long hours at the office, family responsibilities, and other commitments, it's easy for exercise to fall to the bottom of your priority list. However, incorporating exercise into your workday is not only possible but also essential for your overall well-being and productivity. In this section, we will explore practical strategies to help you seamlessly integrate exercise into your daily routine.

1. Prioritize Movement Breaks

One of the simplest ways to incorporate exercise into your workday is by prioritizing movement breaks. Instead of sitting at your desk for hours on end, make it a habit to take short breaks throughout the day to move your body. This could involve stretching, walking around the office, or even doing a quick workout routine. Not only will these breaks help you stay physically active, but they will also boost your energy levels and improve your focus.

2. Make Use of Your Commute

For many working women, commuting to and from work takes up a significant portion of their day. Instead of viewing this time as wasted, consider using it as an opportunity to incorporate exercise. If possible, try walking or biking to work instead of driving or taking public transportation. If walking or biking isn't feasible, you can still make use of your commute by parking farther away from your office or getting off the bus or train a few stops earlier and walking the rest of the way.

3. Schedule Active Meetings

Rather than always sitting in a conference room for meetings, consider scheduling active meetings whenever appropriate. This could involve taking a walk with your colleagues while discussing work-related matters or even holding standing meetings. Not only will these active meetings help you get some exercise, but they can also foster creativity and collaboration among team members.

4. Desk Exercises and Stretches

When you're stuck at your desk for long periods, desk exercises and stretches can be a lifesaver. Simple exercises like leg lifts, desk push-ups, or seated twists can help you stay active and prevent stiffness and muscle tension. Additionally, incorporating stretching breaks into your workday can help improve your flexibility and reduce the risk of injuries.

5. Utilize Fitness Apps and Online Workouts

In today's digital age, there are countless fitness apps and online workout platforms available that cater to busy individuals. These apps and platforms offer a wide range of workouts that can be done in a short amount of time and require minimal equipment. Whether it's a 10-minute yoga session or a high-intensity interval training (HIIT) workout, you can easily find options that fit your schedule and fitness level. Consider downloading a fitness app or subscribing to an online workout platform to have access to a variety of exercises that you can do during your lunch break or whenever you have a few minutes to spare.

6. Create a Lunchtime Routine

Instead of spending your lunch break sitting at your desk or grabbing a quick bite to eat, use this time to prioritize your health and well-being. Create a lunchtime routine that includes physical activity, such as going for a walk, attending a fitness class, or doing a quick workout. Not only will this help you incorporate exercise into your workday, but it will also provide a much-needed mental break and boost your productivity for the rest of the day.

7. Encourage Workplace Wellness Programs

If your workplace doesn't already have a wellness program in place, consider advocating for one. Workplace wellness programs can include initiatives such as fitness challenges, group exercise classes, or even access to an on-site gym. By encouraging your employer to prioritize employee health and well-being, you can create an environment that supports and promotes exercise during the workday.

8. Stay Active During Breaks

Instead of spending your coffee or tea breaks scrolling through social media or chatting with colleagues, use this time to get moving. Take a brisk walk around the office, climb a few flights of stairs, or do a quick set of exercises. These short bursts of activity can add up throughout the day and help you meet your daily exercise goals.

9. Set Reminders and Accountability

Incorporating exercise into your workday requires consistency and commitment. Set reminders on your phone or computer to prompt you to take movement breaks or engage in physical activity. Additionally, find an accountability partner, whether it's a colleague, friend, or family member, who can help keep you motivated and on track with your exercise goals.

Remember, the key to incorporating exercise into your workday is to make it a priority and find creative ways to fit it into your schedule. By prioritizing movement breaks, utilizing your commute, scheduling active meetings, and making use of fitness apps and online workouts, you can seamlessly integrate exercise into your daily routine. With a little planning and determination, you can achieve a healthy work-life balance and reap the numerous benefits of regular exercise.

2.4 Overcoming Obstacles and Excuses

As a working woman, it's common to face obstacles and make excuses when it comes to balancing work and fitness. However, it's important to remember that these obstacles and excuses can be overcome with the right mindset and strategies. In this section, we will explore some common obstacles and excuses and provide practical tips to help you overcome them.

Lack of Time

One of the most common obstacles for working women when it comes to exercise is a lack of time. Between work responsibilities, household chores, and family commitments, finding time for fitness can seem impossible. However, it's essential to prioritize your health and make time for exercise.

Here are some strategies to overcome the lack of time:

1. **Schedule your workouts**: Treat your exercise time as an important appointment and schedule it in your calendar. By setting aside specific time slots for exercise, you are more likely to follow through.

2. **Break it up**: If finding a continuous block of time for exercise is challenging, break your workouts into shorter sessions throughout the day. For example, you can do a 15-minute workout in the morning, another 15 minutes during your lunch break, and a final 15 minutes in the evening.

3. **Multitask**: Look for opportunities to incorporate exercise into your daily routine. For instance, you can do squats or lunges while brushing your teeth, take the stairs instead of the elevator, or go for a walk during your lunch break.

Lack of Energy

Feeling tired and lacking energy after a long day of work is a common excuse for skipping exercise. However, regular physical activity can actually boost your energy levels and improve your overall well-being. Overcoming this excuse requires a shift in mindset and some practical strategies.

Here are some tips to overcome the lack of energy:

1. **Start small**: On days when you feel low on energy, start with a shorter and less intense workout. Even a 10-minute walk or a gentle yoga session can help you feel more energized.

2. **Choose the right time**: Pay attention to your energy levels throughout the day and identify the time when you feel most energized. Schedule your workouts during these peak energy periods to make the most of your exercise sessions.

3. **Fuel your body**: Ensure that you are eating a balanced diet and staying hydrated throughout the day. Proper nutrition and hydration play a crucial role in maintaining energy levels. Consider having a light snack before your workout to provide an extra boost of energy.

Lack of Motivation

Finding motivation to exercise can be challenging, especially after a long day at work. However, it's important to remember your goals and the benefits of regular physical activity. Overcoming the lack of motivation requires finding strategies that work for you and keeping your goals in mind.

Here are some strategies to overcome the lack of motivation:

1. **Set realistic goals**: Break down your fitness goals into smaller, achievable milestones. Celebrate your progress along the way to stay motivated and focused.

2. **Find an accountability partner**: Partnering with a friend or colleague who shares similar fitness goals can provide the motivation and support you need. You can hold each other accountable and even work out together.

3. **Mix it up**: Trying new activities and workouts can help keep your exercise routine exciting and prevent boredom. Explore different fitness classes, outdoor activities, or online workout programs to find what you enjoy the most.

Feeling Overwhelmed

Balancing work and fitness can sometimes feel overwhelming, especially when you have a lot on your plate. However, it's important to remember that self-care, including exercise, is essential for your overall well-being. Overcoming this feeling of overwhelm requires prioritization and effective time management.

Here are some tips to overcome feeling overwhelmed:

1. **Delegate and ask for help**: Don't be afraid to delegate tasks at work or at home. Ask for help from your colleagues, family members, or friends to lighten your load and create more time for exercise.

2. **Practice self-care**: Taking care of yourself is not selfish; it's necessary. Prioritize self-care activities such as exercise, meditation, or relaxation techniques to reduce stress and improve your overall well-being.

3. **Break it down**: When you have a lot on your plate, break your tasks into smaller, manageable chunks. Focus on one task at a time and avoid multitasking, as it can lead to increased stress and decreased productivity.

Remember, overcoming obstacles and excuses requires commitment and a positive mindset. By prioritizing your health and making exercise a non-negotiable part of your routine, you can overcome any obstacle that comes your way. Stay focused on your goals, stay motivated, and remember that you have the power to balance work and fitness successfully.

Nutrition for Optimal Performance

3.1 Understanding the Role of Nutrition

Nutrition plays a crucial role in our overall health and well-being. It provides our bodies with the necessary nutrients, vitamins, and minerals to function optimally. For working women, understanding the role of nutrition is essential for maintaining energy levels, supporting physical activity, and promoting overall wellness.

The Basics of Nutrition

Nutrition is the process by which our bodies obtain and utilize the nutrients needed for growth, repair, and maintenance. These nutrients include carbohydrates, proteins, fats, vitamins, minerals, and water. Each of these components plays a unique role in our bodies and has specific functions.

Carbohydrates are the body's primary source of energy. They provide fuel for our muscles and brain, allowing us to perform daily tasks and exercise. Good sources of carbohydrates include whole grains, fruits, vegetables, and legumes.

Proteins are essential for building and repairing tissues, as well as supporting the immune system. They are made up of amino acids, which are the building blocks of our bodies. Good sources of protein include lean meats, poultry, fish, eggs, dairy products, legumes, and nuts.

Fats are important for providing energy, insulating and protecting organs, and aiding in the absorption of fat-soluble vitamins. It is important to choose healthy fats, such as those found in avocados, nuts, seeds, olive oil, and fatty fish, while limiting saturated and trans fats.

Vitamins and minerals are micronutrients that are necessary for various bodily functions. They help support our immune system, maintain healthy bones and teeth, and assist in the production of energy. Fruits, vegetables, whole grains, and lean proteins are excellent sources of vitamins and minerals.

Water is often overlooked but is vital for our bodies to function properly. It helps regulate body temperature, aids in digestion, transports nutrients, and flushes out waste products. It is recommended to drink at least eight glasses of water per day, or more if you are physically active or in a hot climate.

The Impact of Nutrition on Energy and Endurance

As a working woman, you need sustained energy throughout the day to meet the demands of your job and maintain an active lifestyle. Proper nutrition plays a significant role in providing the energy needed for both mental and physical tasks.

Carbohydrates are the body's preferred source of energy. When consumed, they are broken down into glucose, which is used by our cells for energy. Including complex carbohydrates, such as whole grains, fruits, and vegetables, in your meals and snacks can help provide a steady release of energy throughout the day.

Protein is also important for energy and endurance. It helps repair and build muscle tissue, which is especially beneficial for women who engage in regular exercise. Including lean sources of protein, such as chicken, fish, tofu, or beans, in your meals can help support muscle recovery and provide sustained energy.

Fats, particularly healthy fats, are another source of energy. They are more calorie-dense than carbohydrates and proteins, providing a concentrated source of fuel. Including small amounts of healthy fats, such as avocado, nuts, or olive oil, in your meals can help provide a feeling of satiety and sustained energy.

Hydration is crucial for maintaining energy levels and endurance. Dehydration can lead to fatigue, decreased cognitive function, and reduced physical performance. Make sure to drink water throughout the day, especially during and after exercise, to stay properly hydrated.

The Importance of Balanced Meals and Snacks

To maintain optimal energy levels and support physical activity, it is important to focus on balanced meals and snacks. A balanced meal consists of a combination of carbohydrates, proteins, and fats, along with a variety of fruits and vegetables.

Start by including a source of lean protein in each meal, such as chicken, fish, tofu, or beans. Protein helps keep you feeling full and satisfied, and it supports muscle recovery and growth.

Next, include a serving of complex carbohydrates, such as whole grains, fruits, or starchy vegetables. These provide a steady release of energy and help fuel your brain and muscles.

Don't forget to include healthy fats in your meals as well. These can come from sources like avocados, nuts, seeds, or olive oil. Fats help provide satiety and support the absorption of fat-soluble vitamins.

Lastly, fill your plate with a variety of colorful fruits and vegetables. These provide essential vitamins, minerals, and antioxidants that support overall health and well-being.

In addition to balanced meals, incorporating healthy snacks throughout the day can help maintain energy levels and prevent overeating. Opt for snacks that combine protein, carbohydrates, and healthy fats, such as Greek yogurt with berries, a handful of nuts and seeds, or a piece of fruit with nut butter.

The Role of Nutrition in Weight Management

Proper nutrition is also essential for weight management. As a working woman, finding a healthy balance between work and fitness can be challenging, but understanding the role of nutrition can greatly support your weight management goals.

Maintaining a calorie balance is key to weight management. Consuming more calories than your body needs can lead to weight gain, while consuming fewer calories can lead to weight loss. It is important to find a balance that supports your energy needs and goals.

Incorporating nutrient-dense foods, such as fruits, vegetables, whole grains, lean proteins, and healthy fats, into your meals and snacks can help you feel satisfied while providing essential nutrients. These foods are typically lower in calories and higher in fiber, which can help promote feelings of fullness.

Portion control is another important aspect of weight management. Paying attention to portion sizes and practicing mindful eating can help prevent overeating. It can be helpful to use measuring cups or a food scale to ensure you are consuming appropriate portions.

Additionally, being mindful of your eating habits and emotions can support healthy weight management. Emotional eating or eating out of boredom can lead to consuming excess calories. Finding alternative ways to cope with stress or emotions, such as engaging in physical activity or practicing relaxation techniques, can help prevent emotional eating.

Understanding the role of nutrition in weight management is crucial for achieving and maintaining a healthy weight. By focusing on balanced meals, portion control, and mindful eating, you can support your weight management goals while maintaining energy levels for work and fitness.

In conclusion, nutrition plays a vital role in the lives of working women. Understanding the basics of nutrition, its impact on energy and endurance, the importance of balanced meals and snacks, and its role in weight management can empower you to make informed choices that support your overall health and well-being. By prioritizing nutrition and making conscious decisions about what you eat, you can fuel your body for success in both your professional and fitness endeavors.

3.2 Eating for Energy and Endurance

As a busy working woman, it's essential to fuel your body with the right nutrients to maintain energy and endurance throughout the day. Proper nutrition plays a crucial role in supporting your physical and mental well-being, allowing you to perform at your best both at work and during your workouts. In this section, we will explore the importance of eating for energy and endurance and provide practical tips to help you make healthy food choices.

The Role of Nutrition in Energy and Endurance

Nutrition is the foundation of optimal performance, whether it's at work or during exercise. The food you consume directly impacts your energy levels, focus, and overall stamina. By understanding the role of nutrition in energy and endurance, you can make informed choices to support your body's needs.

Macronutrients for Energy Macronutrients, including carbohydrates, proteins, and fats, are the primary sources of energy for your body. Carbohydrates are especially important as they provide the quickest and most readily available source of fuel. Incorporating complex carbohydrates like whole grains, fruits, and vegetables into your meals can provide sustained energy throughout the day.

Proteins are essential for muscle repair and growth, which is crucial for endurance and strength. Include lean sources of protein such as chicken, fish, tofu, and legumes in your meals to support your body's recovery and maintenance.

Healthy fats, such as those found in avocados, nuts, and olive oil, are also important for energy and endurance. They provide a concentrated source of energy and help regulate hormone production, which is vital for overall well-being.

Micronutrients for Endurance In addition to macronutrients, micronutrients play a crucial role in supporting endurance and overall health. Micronutrients include vitamins and minerals that are essential for various bodily functions. Some key micronutrients for endurance include:

- Iron: Iron is necessary for the production of red blood cells, which carry oxygen to your muscles. Include iron-rich foods like lean meats, spinach, and lentils in your diet to prevent fatigue and support endurance.

- B vitamins: B vitamins, including B12 and folate, are involved in energy production and the formation of red blood cells. Incorporate foods like whole grains, leafy greens, and eggs to ensure an adequate intake of B vitamins.

- Magnesium: Magnesium is involved in muscle function and energy metabolism. Foods rich in magnesium include nuts, seeds, leafy greens, and whole grains.

- Antioxidants: Antioxidants, such as vitamins C and E, help protect your cells from oxidative stress caused by intense exercise. Include colorful fruits and vegetables, nuts, and seeds in your diet to boost your antioxidant intake.

Tips for Eating for Energy and Endurance

Now that you understand the importance of nutrition for energy and endurance, let's explore some practical tips to help you make healthy food choices:

1. Eat Balanced Meals Focus on creating balanced meals that include a combination of carbohydrates, proteins, and healthy fats. This will provide your body with a steady release of energy and support muscle recovery. Aim to include a variety of colorful fruits and vegetables to ensure you're getting a wide range of vitamins and minerals.

2. Prioritize Whole Foods Choose whole, unprocessed foods whenever possible. These foods are rich in nutrients and provide sustained energy. Opt for whole grains, lean proteins, and plenty of fruits and vegetables. Avoid processed foods that are high in added sugars, unhealthy fats, and artificial ingredients.

3. Stay Hydrated Dehydration can lead to fatigue and decreased performance. Make sure to drink enough water throughout the day to stay hydrated. Carry a water bottle with you and sip on water regularly, especially during intense workouts or long workdays.

4. Plan and Prepare Meals Meal planning and preparation can save you time and ensure you have nutritious meals readily available. Set aside some time each week to plan your meals, create a shopping list, and prepare meals in advance. This will help you avoid relying on unhealthy takeout options when you're busy or tired.

5. Snack Smartly Choose healthy snacks that provide sustained energy and support your endurance. Opt for snacks that combine carbohydrates and proteins, such as Greek yogurt with berries, a handful of nuts and seeds, or a whole grain wrap with lean protein. Avoid sugary snacks and opt for whole food options instead.

6. Listen to Your Body Pay attention to your body's hunger and fullness cues. Eat when you're hungry and stop when you're satisfied. Avoid restrictive diets or skipping meals, as they can lead to low energy levels and decreased performance.

7. Seek Professional Guidance If you're unsure about your nutritional needs or have specific dietary requirements, consider consulting a registered dietitian or nutritionist. They can provide personalized guidance and help you create a meal plan that supports your energy and endurance goals.

By incorporating these tips into your daily routine, you can optimize your nutrition for energy and endurance. Remember, nourishing your body with the right foods is an investment in your overall well-being and success as a working woman.

3.3 Meal Planning and Prepping

Meal planning and prepping is a crucial aspect of maintaining a healthy and balanced lifestyle, especially for busy working women. When you have a hectic schedule, it can be challenging to find the time and energy to cook nutritious meals every day. However, with a little bit of planning and preparation, you can ensure that you have healthy and delicious meals ready to go, saving you time and helping you stay on track with your fitness goals.

The Benefits of Meal Planning and Prepping

Meal planning and prepping offers numerous benefits for working women. Here are a few reasons why you should consider incorporating this practice into your routine:

1. **Saves time**: By dedicating a specific time each week to plan and prepare your meals, you can save valuable time during the week. Instead of spending hours each day figuring out what to cook and then preparing it, you can simply grab your pre-prepared meals and go.

2. **Promotes healthier choices**: When you plan your meals in advance, you have more control over what you eat. This allows you to make healthier choices and avoid impulsive decisions that may not align with your fitness goals. By having nutritious meals readily available, you are less likely to reach for unhealthy options or rely on takeout.

3. **Reduces stress**: Meal planning and prepping can significantly reduce stress, especially during busy workdays. Knowing that you have a well-balanced meal waiting for you can alleviate the pressure of having to cook after a long day. It also eliminates the need to rush to the grocery store or order takeout, which can be both time-consuming and stressful.

4. **Saves money**: When you plan your meals in advance, you can make a shopping list and buy only the ingredients you need. This helps you avoid unnecessary purchases and reduces food waste. Additionally, by cooking your meals at home, you can save money compared to eating out or ordering takeout regularly.

Getting Started with Meal Planning and Prepping

Now that you understand the benefits, let's dive into how you can get started with meal planning and prepping:

1. **Set aside time for planning**: Dedicate a specific day or time each week to plan your meals. This could be on a Sunday afternoon or any other day that works best for you. Use this time to decide what meals you want to prepare for the upcoming week.

2. **Create a meal plan**: Start by creating a meal plan for the week. Consider your schedule, dietary preferences, and fitness goals when selecting recipes. Aim for a balance of protein, carbohydrates, and healthy fats in each meal. Include a variety of fruits, vegetables, whole grains, and lean proteins to ensure you're getting all the necessary nutrients.

3. **Make a shopping list**: Once you have your meal plan, make a detailed shopping list. Check your pantry and fridge to see what ingredients you already have and only purchase what you need. This will help you stay organized and avoid buying unnecessary items.

4. **Prep ingredients in advance**: After grocery shopping, set aside some time to prep ingredients in advance. Wash and chop vegetables, cook grains, and marinate proteins if needed. This will save you time during the week and make it easier to assemble your meals.

5. **Cook in batches**: Consider cooking larger portions of certain dishes that can be easily reheated or repurposed throughout the week. For example, you can cook a big batch of grilled chicken breast and use it in salads, wraps, or stir-fries. This way, you'll have a variety of meals without having to cook every day.

6. **Store meals properly**: Invest in good quality food storage containers that are microwave and freezer-safe. Portion out your meals and store them in the fridge or freezer, depending on when you plan to consume them. Label each container with the meal and date to keep track of freshness.

7. **Mix and match**: Don't be afraid to mix and match ingredients to create different meals throughout the week. For example, you can use roasted vegetables in salads, wraps, or as a side dish. This adds variety to your meals and prevents boredom.

8. **Stay flexible**: While meal planning and prepping can be incredibly helpful, it's essential to stay flexible. Life happens, and sometimes plans change. Be open to adjusting your meal plan if needed and have backup options available, such as frozen meals or healthy takeout choices.

By following these steps, you can establish a meal planning and prepping routine that works for you. Remember, it may take some trial and error to find the best approach, so don't get discouraged if it doesn't go perfectly at first. With practice, you'll become more efficient and find a system that fits seamlessly into your busy lifestyle.

Tips for Successful Meal Planning and Prepping

To make your meal planning and prepping experience even more successful, consider the following tips:

1. **Keep it simple**: Start with simple recipes that require minimal ingredients and preparation. As you become more comfortable with meal planning and prepping, you can gradually experiment with more complex dishes.

2. **Use versatile ingredients**: Opt for ingredients that can be used in multiple recipes. For example, roasted chicken breast can be added to salads, wraps, or served with roasted vegetables.

3. **Utilize your freezer**: If you have limited fridge space or know that you won't be able to consume all your meals within a few days, freeze them for later use. This allows you to have a variety of meals readily available without worrying about spoilage.

4. **Try theme nights**: Assign specific themes to different days of the week to make meal planning more fun. For example, you can have "Meatless Monday," "Taco Tuesday," or "Stir-Fry Friday." This adds variety and excitement to your meals.

5. **Get the family involved**: If you have a family, involve them in the meal planning and prepping process. This not only lightens your workload but also encourages healthier eating habits for everyone.

6. **Experiment with new recipes**: Don't be afraid to try new recipes and flavors. Use meal planning and prepping as an opportunity to expand your culinary skills and discover new favorite dishes.

Remember, meal planning and prepping is a tool to help you stay on track with your fitness goals and maintain a healthy lifestyle. It's not about perfection but rather finding a system that works for you. With practice and consistency, you'll soon reap the benefits of this time-saving and health-enhancing practice.

3.4 Healthy Snacking at Work

When it comes to maintaining a healthy lifestyle, what you eat plays a crucial role. This is especially true when you're at work, where it can be tempting to reach for unhealthy snacks or indulge in sugary treats. However, with a little planning and preparation, you can make healthy snacking at work a breeze. In this section, we will explore some practical tips and ideas to help you make smart snack choices and keep your energy levels up throughout the day.

3.4.1 The Importance of Healthy Snacking

Snacking is an essential part of maintaining a balanced diet, especially for busy working women. Healthy snacks can provide you with the necessary nutrients and energy to keep you focused and productive throughout the day. They can also help prevent overeating during meals and keep your metabolism running smoothly.

3.4.2 Planning and Preparing Snacks in Advance

One of the keys to successful healthy snacking at work is planning and preparation. By taking a little time to plan and prepare your snacks in advance, you can avoid reaching for unhealthy options when hunger strikes. Here are some tips to help you get started:

1. **Create a snack plan**: Take a few minutes each week to plan out your snacks for the upcoming days. Consider your nutritional needs and choose a variety of snacks that include protein, healthy fats, and fiber.

2. **Stock up on healthy options**: Keep your pantry and desk drawer stocked with nutritious snacks such as nuts, seeds, dried fruits, whole grain crackers, and low-sugar protein bars. Having these options readily available will make it easier to resist the temptation of unhealthy snacks.

3. **Pre-portion your snacks**: To avoid mindlessly eating large quantities of snacks, pre-portion them into individual servings. This will help you control your portion sizes and prevent overeating.

4. **Pack your snacks the night before**: Take a few minutes each evening to pack your snacks for the next day. This way, you won't be rushed in the morning and can ensure you have a variety of healthy options to choose from.

3.4.3 Healthy Snack Ideas for Work

Now that you understand the importance of healthy snacking and how to plan and prepare your snacks, let's explore some delicious and nutritious snack ideas that are perfect for the workplace:

1. **Greek yogurt with berries**: Greek yogurt is packed with protein and calcium, while berries add a burst of antioxidants and fiber. Combine the two for a satisfying and refreshing snack.

2. **Vegetable sticks with hummus**: Cut up some carrot, cucumber, and bell pepper sticks and pair them with a serving of hummus. This snack is not only delicious but also provides a good dose of vitamins, minerals, and healthy fats.

3. **Hard-boiled eggs**: Hard-boiled eggs are a convenient and protein-rich snack option. They are easy to prepare in advance and can be enjoyed on

their own or paired with whole grain crackers.

4. **Homemade trail mix**: Create your own trail mix by combining a variety of nuts, seeds, and dried fruits. This snack is portable, customizable, and provides a good balance of healthy fats, protein, and carbohydrates.

5. **Avocado toast**: Toast a slice of whole grain bread and top it with mashed avocado, a sprinkle of sea salt, and a squeeze of lemon juice. This snack is not only delicious but also provides healthy fats and fiber.

6. **Cottage cheese with fruit**: Cottage cheese is a great source of protein, and when paired with fresh fruit like pineapple or berries, it becomes a tasty and nutritious snack.

7. **Homemade energy balls**: Make a batch of energy balls using ingredients like oats, nut butter, honey, and dried fruits. These bite-sized snacks are packed with energy and can be enjoyed throughout the day.

8. **Roasted chickpeas**: Roast a can of chickpeas with a drizzle of olive oil and your favorite spices for a crunchy and protein-packed snack. They are a great alternative to chips or other unhealthy snacks.

Remember, the key to healthy snacking at work is to choose snacks that are nutrient-dense and provide a good balance of macronutrients. Avoid snacks that are high in added sugars, unhealthy fats, and empty calories.

3.4.4 Tips for Snacking Mindfully

In addition to choosing healthy snacks, it's important to practice mindful eating. Mindful eating involves paying attention to your body's hunger and fullness cues and savoring each bite. Here are some tips to help you snack mindfully at work:

1. **Eat without distractions**: Avoid eating at your desk while working or scrolling through your phone. Instead, find a quiet space where you can focus on your snack and enjoy the flavors and textures.

2. **Take small bites and chew slowly**: Take the time to savor each bite and chew your food thoroughly. This will not only help with digestion but also allow you to fully enjoy the taste of your snack.

3. **Listen to your body**: Pay attention to your body's hunger and fullness signals. Eat when you're hungry and stop when you're satisfied, rather than eating out of boredom or stress.

4. **Practice portion control**: Be mindful of your portion sizes and avoid mindlessly eating large quantities of snacks. Use small bowls or plates to help control your portions.

5. **Engage your senses**: Take a moment to appreciate the colors, smells, and textures of your snack. Engaging your senses can enhance your eating experience and make it more enjoyable.

By practicing mindful eating, you can develop a healthier relationship with food and make more conscious choices when it comes to snacking at work.

Conclusion

Healthy snacking at work is not only possible but also essential for maintaining your energy levels and overall well-being. By planning and preparing your snacks in advance, choosing nutrient-dense options, and practicing mindful eating, you can make smart snack choices that support your work and fitness goals. Remember, small changes in your snacking habits can have a big impact on your health and productivity. So, start incorporating these healthy snack ideas into your work routine and enjoy the benefits of nourishing your body throughout the day.

3.5 Navigating Social and Work Events

As a working woman, it's important to strike a balance between your professional life and your fitness goals. However, social and work events can often throw a wrench into your routine and make it challenging to stay on track. But fear not! With a little planning and preparation, you can navigate these events while still prioritizing your health and fitness.

1. Plan Ahead

One of the keys to successfully navigating social and work events is to plan ahead. Take a look at your calendar and identify any upcoming events that may pose a challenge to your fitness routine. This could be anything from a work conference to a birthday party. Once you have a clear idea of what's coming up, you can start strategizing.

2. Communicate Your Goals

Don't be afraid to communicate your fitness goals to your colleagues, friends, and family. Let them know that you're committed to leading a healthy lifestyle and that you may need their support during social and work events. By sharing your goals, you're more likely to receive understanding and encouragement from those around you.

3. Be Mindful of Your Choices

When attending social and work events, it's important to be mindful of your choices. While it's okay to indulge occasionally, try to make healthier choices whenever possible. Opt for lean proteins, vegetables, and whole grains instead of fried or sugary foods. Choose water or unsweetened beverages over sugary cocktails or sodas. By making conscious choices, you can still enjoy yourself while staying on track with your fitness goals.

4. Bring Your Own Dish

If you're attending a potluck or a gathering where you have the opportunity to bring a dish, take advantage of it. Prepare a healthy and delicious dish that aligns with your fitness goals. Not only will you have a healthy option to enjoy, but you'll also be able to share your commitment to health and fitness with others.

5. Practice Portion Control

Portion control is key when navigating social and work events. It's easy to get carried away with the abundance of food and drinks available. Instead of piling your plate high, take smaller portions and savor each bite. Listen to your body's hunger and fullness cues, and stop eating when you're satisfied. By practicing portion control, you can enjoy the event without overindulging.

6. Be Selective with Alcohol

Alcohol can be a common feature at social and work events, but it's important to be selective with your choices. Alcoholic beverages can be high in calories and can hinder your progress towards your fitness goals. Opt for lighter options like wine or spirits mixed with soda water instead of sugary cocktails or heavy beers. Remember to drink in moderation and stay hydrated by alternating alcoholic beverages with water.

7. Stay Active

Even during social and work events, find ways to stay active. If the event allows, take breaks to stretch or go for a short walk. Engage in conversations while standing or walking around instead of sitting for long periods. If there's a dance floor, don't be afraid to hit it and get your heart rate up. By incorporating movement into these events, you can still get some exercise while enjoying yourself.

8. Seek Support

If you find it challenging to navigate social and work events while staying on track with your fitness goals, seek support from like-minded individuals. Join fitness groups or online communities where you can connect with others who are facing similar challenges. Share your experiences, seek advice, and offer support to one another. Having a support system can make a world of difference in staying motivated and accountable.

9. Practice Mindful Eating

Mindful eating is a powerful tool when it comes to navigating social and work events. Instead of mindlessly indulging in every treat or dish available, take the time to savor and enjoy each bite. Pay attention to the flavors, textures, and sensations of the food. Eat slowly and listen to your body's cues of hunger and fullness. By practicing mindful eating, you can make conscious choices and avoid overeating.

10. Don't Beat Yourself Up

Lastly, it's important to remember that perfection is not the goal. There will be times when you may indulge more than you planned or miss a workout due to a work event. It's okay! Don't beat yourself up over it. Instead, focus on the progress you've made and the healthy habits you've incorporated into your lifestyle. Learn from any setbacks and use them as motivation to continue moving forward.

Navigating social and work events as a working woman can be challenging, but with the right mindset and strategies, it's absolutely possible to stay on track with your fitness goals. Plan ahead, make mindful choices, seek support, and practice self-compassion. Remember, you have the power to prioritize your health and fitness while still enjoying these events to the fullest.

3.6 Fueling Your Body for Exercise

Proper nutrition is essential for fueling your body and maximizing your performance during exercise. As a working woman, it's important to prioritize your nutrition to ensure you have the energy and stamina to tackle your workouts. In this section, we will explore the key principles of fueling your body for exercise and provide practical tips to help you make informed choices about what to eat before, during, and after your workouts.

Understanding the Role of Nutrition

Nutrition plays a crucial role in supporting your exercise routine. It provides the necessary fuel to power your workouts, aids in muscle recovery and repair, and helps maintain overall health and well-being. When it comes to exercise, there are a few key nutrients to focus on:

1. **Carbohydrates**: Carbs are the primary source of energy for your muscles. They are stored as glycogen in your muscles and liver and are readily available for use during exercise. Include complex carbohydrates like whole grains, fruits, and vegetables in your diet to provide sustained energy throughout your workouts.

2. **Protein**: Protein is essential for muscle repair and growth. It helps repair the damage caused by exercise and supports the development of lean muscle mass. Include lean sources of protein such as chicken, fish, tofu, beans, and lentils in your meals and snacks.

3. **Healthy Fats**: While carbohydrates are the primary fuel source for exercise, healthy fats provide a concentrated source of energy and help

regulate hormone production. Include sources of healthy fats like avocados, nuts, seeds, and olive oil in your diet.

4. **Hydration**: Staying hydrated is crucial for optimal exercise performance. Water helps regulate body temperature, lubricates joints, and transports nutrients to your muscles. Aim to drink enough water throughout the day and especially before, during, and after your workouts.

Pre-Workout Nutrition

What you eat before your workout can significantly impact your performance and energy levels. Here are some guidelines to follow when fueling your body before exercise:

1. **Timing**: Aim to eat a balanced meal or snack containing carbohydrates, protein, and a small amount of healthy fats 1-3 hours before your workout. This will give your body enough time to digest and absorb the nutrients.

2. **Carbohydrates**: Prioritize complex carbohydrates like whole grains, fruits, and vegetables. They provide a steady release of energy and help sustain your workout intensity.

3. **Protein**: Include a moderate amount of protein to support muscle repair and growth. This can come from sources like Greek yogurt, eggs, or a protein shake.

4. **Hydration**: Drink water before your workout to ensure you are adequately hydrated. If you're engaging in intense or prolonged exercise, consider a sports drink that contains electrolytes to replenish lost fluids.

Sample pre-workout meal ideas include a whole grain toast with peanut butter and banana, a chicken and vegetable stir-fry with brown rice, or a smoothie with Greek yogurt, berries, and spinach.

During-Workout Nutrition

For shorter workouts, you may not need to consume additional calories during your exercise session. However, for longer or more intense workouts, it may be beneficial to provide your body with some fuel to sustain your energy levels. Here are some tips for during-workout nutrition:

1. **Hydration**: Drink water or a sports drink to stay hydrated during your workout. Sip on fluids regularly, especially if you're sweating heavily.

2. **Carbohydrates**: If your workout exceeds 60-90 minutes, consider consuming easily digestible carbohydrates to maintain your energy levels. Options include energy gels, sports drinks, or small snacks like a banana or a handful of raisins.

3. **Electrolytes**: If you're engaging in prolonged exercise or sweating heavily, consider consuming electrolytes to replenish what you've lost. Electrolyte

tablets or sports drinks can help maintain proper hydration and electrolyte balance.

Remember to listen to your body and adjust your nutrition strategy based on the duration and intensity of your workouts. Experiment with different options to find what works best for you.

Post-Workout Nutrition

After your workout, it's crucial to replenish your body with the nutrients it needs to recover and repair. Here are some guidelines for post-workout nutrition:

1. **Timing**: Aim to consume a balanced meal or snack containing carbohydrates and protein within 30-60 minutes after your workout. This window is known as the "anabolic window" when your body is most receptive to nutrient absorption.

2. **Carbohydrates**: Include carbohydrates to replenish glycogen stores and provide energy for muscle recovery. Opt for complex carbohydrates like sweet potatoes, quinoa, or whole grain bread.

3. **Protein**: Consume a moderate amount of protein to support muscle repair and growth. Lean sources of protein like chicken, fish, tofu, or a protein shake are excellent options.

4. **Hydration**: Drink water to rehydrate your body after exercise. If you've engaged in intense or prolonged exercise, consider a sports drink to replenish electrolytes.

Sample post-workout meal ideas include a grilled chicken salad with quinoa, roasted vegetables with tofu, or a protein smoothie with spinach, banana, and almond milk.

Individualized Approach

It's important to remember that everyone's nutritional needs may vary based on factors such as body composition, exercise intensity, and personal goals. Experiment with different foods and strategies to find what works best for you. Consider consulting with a registered dietitian or nutritionist who can provide personalized guidance based on your specific needs and preferences.

By fueling your body with the right nutrients before, during, and after exercise, you can optimize your performance, enhance your recovery, and achieve your fitness goals as a working woman. Remember to prioritize hydration, include a balance of carbohydrates and protein, and listen to your body's cues. With a well-fueled body, you'll be ready to conquer any workout that comes your way.

Mindset and Mental Health

4.1 The Connection Between Mind and Body

In today's fast-paced world, it's easy for women to get caught up in the hustle and bustle of work and forget to take care of themselves. However, it's important to recognize the strong connection between the mind and body and how they both play a crucial role in our overall well-being. In this section, we will explore the connection between the mind and body and discuss strategies to maintain a healthy balance.

The Mind-Body Connection

The mind and body are not separate entities but rather interconnected and interdependent. Our thoughts, emotions, and beliefs can have a profound impact on our physical health, and vice versa. When we experience stress, anxiety, or negative emotions, our bodies often respond with physical symptoms such as headaches, muscle tension, or digestive issues. On the other hand, when we engage in activities that promote relaxation and positive thinking, our bodies respond by releasing endorphins and reducing stress hormones.

The Impact of Stress and Anxiety

Stress and anxiety are common experiences in the modern workplace, and they can take a toll on both our mental and physical health. Chronic stress can lead to a weakened immune system, increased risk of cardiovascular disease, and even mental health disorders such as depression. It's crucial to recognize the signs of stress and anxiety and take proactive steps to manage them.

Managing Stress and Anxiety

There are various strategies you can incorporate into your daily routine to manage stress and anxiety effectively:

1. **Exercise**: Engaging in regular physical activity is one of the most effective ways to reduce stress and anxiety. Exercise releases endorphins, which are natural mood boosters, and helps to alleviate tension in the body. Find activities that you enjoy, whether it's going for a run, practicing yoga, or dancing, and make time for them regularly.

2. **Mindfulness and Meditation**: Practicing mindfulness and meditation can help calm the mind and reduce stress. Take a few minutes each day to sit quietly, focus on your breath, and observe your thoughts without judgment. This practice can help you develop a greater sense of self-awareness and improve your ability to manage stress.

3. **Deep Breathing**: Deep breathing exercises can activate the body's relaxation response and help reduce anxiety. Take slow, deep breaths,

inhaling through your nose and exhaling through your mouth. Focus on filling your belly with air and releasing any tension as you exhale.

4. **Time Management**: Poor time management can contribute to feelings of stress and overwhelm. Take the time to prioritize your tasks and create a schedule that allows for breaks and self-care. Delegate tasks when possible and learn to say no to additional responsibilities that may cause unnecessary stress.

5. **Self-Care**: Engaging in activities that bring you joy and relaxation is essential for managing stress. Whether it's taking a bubble bath, reading a book, or spending time in nature, make self-care a priority in your daily routine.

Building Resilience and Confidence

Building resilience and confidence is crucial for maintaining a healthy mind-body connection. Resilience allows us to bounce back from setbacks and challenges, while confidence empowers us to take on new opportunities and overcome self-doubt. Here are some strategies to help you build resilience and confidence:

1. **Positive Self-Talk**: Pay attention to your inner dialogue and replace negative self-talk with positive affirmations. Remind yourself of your strengths and accomplishments, and believe in your ability to overcome challenges.

2. **Set Realistic Goals**: Setting realistic goals and breaking them down into smaller, achievable steps can boost your confidence and motivation. Celebrate each milestone along the way and acknowledge your progress.

3. **Seek Support**: Surround yourself with a supportive network of friends, family, or colleagues who uplift and encourage you. Share your goals and challenges with them, and lean on them for support when needed.

4. **Embrace Failure as a Learning Opportunity**: Failure is a natural part of life, and it's important to view it as a learning opportunity rather than a reflection of your worth. Embrace failure as a chance to grow, learn, and improve.

Practicing Mindfulness and Meditation

Mindfulness and meditation are powerful practices that can help you cultivate a deeper connection between your mind and body. By bringing your attention to the present moment and observing your thoughts and sensations without judgment, you can develop a greater sense of self-awareness and improve your overall well-being. Here are some tips to help you incorporate mindfulness and meditation into your daily routine:

1. **Start Small**: Begin with just a few minutes of mindfulness or meditation each day and gradually increase the duration as you become more com-

fortable. Consistency is key, so aim to practice every day, even if it's just for a few minutes.

2. **Find a Quiet Space**: Choose a quiet and comfortable space where you can sit or lie down without distractions. This could be a corner of your home, a park, or even your office during a break.

3. **Focus on Your Breath**: Use your breath as an anchor to bring your attention to the present moment. Notice the sensation of the breath entering and leaving your body, and let go of any thoughts or distractions that arise.

4. **Explore Guided Meditations**: If you're new to meditation, guided meditations can be a helpful tool. There are many apps and online resources available that offer guided meditations for various purposes, such as stress reduction, sleep, or self-compassion.

Remember, the mind and body are interconnected, and taking care of one is essential for the well-being of the other. By incorporating strategies to manage stress, build resilience, and practice mindfulness, you can strengthen the mind-body connection and achieve a greater sense of balance in your life.

4.2 Managing Stress and Anxiety

In today's fast-paced and demanding world, stress and anxiety have become common experiences for many working women. The pressure to excel in our careers, maintain a healthy work-life balance, and meet societal expectations can often leave us feeling overwhelmed and anxious. However, it is essential to prioritize our mental well-being and develop effective strategies to manage stress and anxiety. In this section, we will explore various techniques and practices that can help you navigate through stressful situations and promote a sense of calm and balance in your life.

Understanding Stress and Anxiety

Before we delve into managing stress and anxiety, it is crucial to understand what these terms mean and how they affect our lives. Stress is the body's response to a perceived threat or demand, whether it is physical, emotional, or psychological. It triggers the release of stress hormones, such as cortisol, which can have both short-term and long-term effects on our health.

Anxiety, on the other hand, is a feeling of unease, worry, or fear about future events or uncertain situations. It can manifest as physical symptoms like a racing heart, shortness of breath, or a knot in the stomach. While stress is often a response to external pressures, anxiety can arise from internal thoughts and concerns.

Identifying Sources of Stress

To effectively manage stress and anxiety, it is essential to identify the sources or triggers that contribute to these feelings. Take some time to reflect on the aspects of your work and personal life that cause you stress. It could be tight deadlines, a heavy workload, conflicts with colleagues, or even personal responsibilities outside of work.

Once you have identified the sources of stress, you can begin to develop strategies to address them. This may involve setting boundaries, delegating tasks, or seeking support from colleagues, friends, or family members. Remember, it is okay to ask for help and prioritize your well-being.

Practicing Stress Management Techniques

There are various stress management techniques that you can incorporate into your daily routine to help reduce stress and anxiety. Here are a few effective strategies:

1. **Deep Breathing**: Deep breathing exercises can help activate the body's relaxation response and calm the mind. Take slow, deep breaths, inhaling through your nose and exhaling through your mouth. Focus on your breath and let go of any tension or worries with each exhale.

2. **Physical Activity**: Engaging in regular physical activity, such as exercise or yoga, can help reduce stress and improve your overall well-being. Find activities that you enjoy and make time for them in your schedule. Even a short walk during your lunch break can have a positive impact on your mood and stress levels.

3. **Mindfulness and Meditation**: Practicing mindfulness and meditation can help you cultivate a sense of present-moment awareness and reduce anxiety. Set aside a few minutes each day to sit quietly, focus on your breath, and observe your thoughts without judgment. There are also many mindfulness apps and guided meditation resources available to assist you in developing a regular practice.

4. **Time Management**: Effective time management can significantly reduce stress levels. Prioritize your tasks, break them down into smaller, manageable steps, and create a schedule or to-do list. This will help you stay organized, avoid procrastination, and create a sense of control over your workload.

5. **Self-Care**: Taking care of yourself is crucial for managing stress and anxiety. Make time for activities that bring you joy and relaxation, such as reading, taking a bath, practicing a hobby, or spending time with loved ones. Prioritize self-care as an essential part of your routine, rather than viewing it as a luxury.

6. **Positive Self-Talk**: Pay attention to your inner dialogue and replace negative self-talk with positive affirmations. Remind yourself of your strengths, accomplishments, and the progress you have made. Cultivating a positive mindset can help reduce stress and increase resilience.

Seeking Professional Support

If stress and anxiety persist despite your efforts to manage them, it may be beneficial to seek professional support. A therapist or counselor can provide guidance and help you develop personalized strategies to cope with stress and anxiety. They can also assist in identifying any underlying issues that may be contributing to your feelings of stress and anxiety.

Remember, managing stress and anxiety is an ongoing process, and what works for one person may not work for another. Be patient with yourself and experiment with different techniques until you find what resonates with you. By prioritizing your mental well-being and implementing effective stress management strategies, you can create a healthier and more balanced life.

4.3 Building Resilience and Confidence

In today's fast-paced and demanding world, building resilience and confidence is essential for every working woman. Resilience refers to the ability to bounce back from setbacks and challenges, while confidence is the belief in oneself and one's abilities. By developing these qualities, you can navigate the ups and downs of work and life with grace and strength. In this section, we will explore strategies and techniques to help you build resilience and confidence.

Embrace a Growth Mindset

One of the first steps in building resilience and confidence is adopting a growth mindset. A growth mindset is the belief that your abilities and intelligence can be developed through dedication and hard work. By embracing this mindset, you can view challenges as opportunities for growth and learning rather than as obstacles.

To cultivate a growth mindset, start by reframing your thoughts and self-talk. Instead of saying, "I can't do this," replace it with, "I can't do this yet, but I'm willing to learn and improve." Celebrate your efforts and progress, even if they are small. Remember that setbacks and failures are part of the learning process and can ultimately lead to success.

Set Realistic Goals

Setting realistic goals is crucial for building resilience and confidence. When you set goals that are attainable and aligned with your values and abilities, you are more likely to experience success and feel confident in your abilities. Start by breaking down your larger goals into smaller, manageable steps. This will not only make them less overwhelming but also allow you to track your progress along the way.

Additionally, it's important to set goals that are within your control. While external factors may influence your progress, focusing on what you can control will help you maintain a sense of resilience and confidence. Remember to celebrate your achievements, no matter how small they may seem. Each step forward is a testament to your resilience and determination.

Practice Self-Compassion

Self-compassion is a powerful tool for building resilience and confidence. It involves treating yourself with kindness, understanding, and acceptance, especially during challenging times. Instead of being overly critical or judgmental, practice self-compassion by offering yourself the same support and encouragement you would give to a friend.

When faced with setbacks or failures, remind yourself that everyone makes mistakes and experiences difficulties. Treat yourself with empathy and understanding, and remember that these experiences are opportunities for growth and learning. By practicing self-compassion, you can build resilience and bounce back from challenges with greater ease.

Cultivate a Supportive Network

Building resilience and confidence is not a journey you have to undertake alone. Cultivating a supportive network of friends, family, and colleagues can provide you with the encouragement and support you need during challenging times. Surround yourself with people who believe in you and your abilities, and who will lift you up when you need it most.

Seek out mentors or role models who have faced similar challenges and have successfully overcome them. Their stories and guidance can inspire and motivate you to persevere. Additionally, consider joining professional or community groups where you can connect with like-minded individuals who share your goals and aspirations. Together, you can support and uplift each other on your journeys.

Practice Self-Care

Taking care of yourself is essential for building resilience and confidence. Self-care involves prioritizing your physical, mental, and emotional well-being. Make time for activities that bring you joy and relaxation, such as exercise, hobbies, or spending time with loved ones. Engage in practices that promote mindfulness and stress reduction, such as meditation or journaling.

Ensure that you are getting enough restful sleep, eating nutritious meals, and staying hydrated. When you prioritize self-care, you are better equipped to handle challenges and setbacks with resilience and confidence. Remember that self-care is not selfish; it is a necessary investment in your overall well-being.

Challenge Yourself

Building resilience and confidence requires stepping outside of your comfort zone and taking on new challenges. By pushing yourself to try new things and take risks, you can expand your skills and capabilities. Start by identifying areas where you feel less confident and set goals to improve in those areas.

Take on projects or tasks that stretch your abilities and require you to learn and grow. Embrace the mindset that failure is not a reflection of your worth but an opportunity for growth. Each time you face a challenge head-on and overcome it, your resilience and confidence will grow stronger.

Practice Positive Self-Talk

The way you talk to yourself has a significant impact on your resilience and confidence. Practice positive self-talk by replacing negative or self-defeating thoughts with positive and empowering ones. Instead of focusing on your weaknesses or past failures, remind yourself of your strengths and past successes.

Affirmations can be a powerful tool for building resilience and confidence. Create a list of positive affirmations that resonate with you and repeat them daily. For example, "I am capable and resilient," or "I have the skills and knowledge to overcome any challenge." By consistently reinforcing positive beliefs about yourself, you can build resilience and confidence from within.

Seek Professional Support

If you find that building resilience and confidence is particularly challenging, consider seeking professional support. A therapist or coach can provide you with guidance and strategies tailored to your specific needs. They can help you identify and overcome any underlying beliefs or patterns that may be hindering your progress.

Remember that seeking help is a sign of strength, not weakness. Professional support can provide you with the tools and resources you need to build resilience and confidence in a supportive and non-judgmental environment.

Building resilience and confidence is a lifelong journey. It requires consistent effort, self-reflection, and a willingness to face challenges head-on. By embracing a growth mindset, setting realistic goals, practicing self-compassion, cultivating a supportive network, and prioritizing self-care, you can build the resilience and confidence needed to thrive in both your work and personal life. Remember, you have the power to overcome any obstacle and achieve your goals.

4.4 Practicing Mindfulness and Meditation

In today's fast-paced world, it's easy for working women to get caught up in the hustle and bustle of everyday life. Between juggling work responsibilities, family commitments, and personal goals, it can feel overwhelming and exhausting.

That's why it's essential for women to prioritize their mental well-being and incorporate mindfulness and meditation practices into their daily routine.

The Power of Mindfulness

Mindfulness is the practice of being fully present in the moment, without judgment or attachment to thoughts or emotions. It involves paying attention to your thoughts, feelings, and sensations in a non-reactive way. By cultivating mindfulness, you can develop a greater sense of self-awareness and improve your ability to manage stress and anxiety.

One of the key benefits of mindfulness is its ability to help you stay focused and engaged in your work. When you practice mindfulness, you train your mind to stay present and avoid getting caught up in distractions or negative thought patterns. This can lead to increased productivity, better decision-making, and improved overall job satisfaction.

Getting Started with Mindfulness

If you're new to mindfulness, it's important to start small and gradually build up your practice. Here are a few simple steps to help you get started:

1. Find a quiet space: Choose a quiet and comfortable space where you can sit or lie down without any distractions.

2. Set a timer: Start with just a few minutes and gradually increase the duration as you become more comfortable with the practice.

3. Focus on your breath: Close your eyes and bring your attention to your breath. Notice the sensation of the breath entering and leaving your body.

4. Notice your thoughts: As you focus on your breath, thoughts will inevitably arise. Instead of getting caught up in them, simply observe them without judgment and gently bring your attention back to your breath.

5. Practice regularly: Consistency is key when it comes to mindfulness. Aim to practice for a few minutes each day, gradually increasing the duration as you progress.

The Benefits of Meditation

Meditation is a powerful tool for reducing stress, improving focus, and promoting overall well-being. It involves training your mind to achieve a state of deep relaxation and heightened awareness. Regular meditation practice can help you cultivate a sense of inner peace and resilience, allowing you to navigate the challenges of work and life with greater ease.

Here are some of the key benefits of incorporating meditation into your daily routine:

1. Stress reduction: Meditation has been shown to reduce the production of stress hormones and activate the body's relaxation response. This can help you manage work-related stress and prevent burnout.

2. Improved focus and concentration: Regular meditation practice can enhance your ability to stay focused and concentrate on tasks, leading to increased productivity and efficiency.

3. Emotional well-being: Meditation can help you develop a greater sense of emotional stability and resilience. It can also improve your ability to regulate emotions and respond to challenging situations with calmness and clarity.

4. Enhanced creativity: By quieting the mind and allowing space for new ideas to emerge, meditation can boost your creativity and problem-solving skills.

Getting Started with Meditation

If you're new to meditation, here are some tips to help you get started:

1. Find a comfortable position: You can sit on a cushion or chair with your back straight, or even lie down if that's more comfortable for you.

2. Choose a focus: You can focus on your breath, a specific word or phrase (known as a mantra), or a visual object. The key is to choose something that helps anchor your attention.

3. Start with a few minutes: Begin with just a few minutes of meditation and gradually increase the duration as you become more comfortable with the practice.

4. Be patient and non-judgmental: It's normal for your mind to wander during meditation. When you notice your thoughts drifting, gently bring your attention back to your chosen focus without judgment.

5. Practice regularly: Consistency is key when it comes to meditation. Aim to practice for at least a few minutes each day, gradually increasing the duration as you progress.

Incorporating Mindfulness and Meditation into Your Workday

Finding time for mindfulness and meditation can be challenging, especially when you have a busy work schedule. However, with a little creativity and intention, you can easily incorporate these practices into your daily routine. Here are some strategies to help you get started:

1. Start your day with mindfulness: Begin your day by setting aside a few minutes for mindfulness practice. This can help you start your day with a clear and focused mind.

2. Take mindful breaks: Throughout the day, take short breaks to practice mindfulness. This can be as simple as taking a few deep breaths, stretching, or going for a short walk outside.

3. Create a meditation space: Designate a quiet corner in your office or home where you can meditate. Decorate it with calming elements such as plants, candles, or soft lighting to create a peaceful atmosphere.

4. Use mindfulness apps: There are many smartphone apps available that offer guided meditations and mindfulness exercises. These can be a great resource for incorporating mindfulness into your workday.

Remember, practicing mindfulness and meditation is a journey, and it's important to be patient and kind to yourself as you develop your practice. With consistent effort and dedication, you can reap the numerous benefits of these practices and find greater balance and well-being in your work and personal life.

Workout Strategies for Busy Women

5.1 Choosing the Right Workout for You

When it comes to incorporating exercise into your busy schedule, choosing the right workout is essential. With so many options available, it can be overwhelming to decide which type of exercise is best for you. However, by considering your goals, preferences, and lifestyle, you can find a workout routine that fits seamlessly into your life. In this section, we will explore different factors to consider when choosing the right workout for you.

Assess Your Goals and Priorities

Before diving into any exercise routine, it's important to assess your goals and priorities. Are you looking to lose weight, build strength, improve cardiovascular fitness, or simply maintain a healthy lifestyle? Understanding your goals will help you narrow down the types of workouts that align with your objectives.

Consider your priorities as well. As a busy working woman, time may be limited, so finding a workout that is efficient and effective is crucial. Additionally, consider your preferences. Do you enjoy high-intensity workouts, or do you prefer something more low-impact and relaxing? By understanding your goals, priorities, and preferences, you can choose a workout that you will enjoy and stick to in the long run.

Explore Different Types of Workouts

There are countless types of workouts available, each offering unique benefits and experiences. Here are a few popular options to consider:

1. **Cardiovascular Exercise**: Cardio workouts, such as running, cycling, or dancing, are great for improving cardiovascular health, burning calories,

and boosting your mood. If you enjoy activities that get your heart rate up and make you break a sweat, cardio exercises may be the perfect fit for you.

2. **Strength Training**: Strength training involves using resistance, such as weights or resistance bands, to build muscle and increase strength. This type of workout is essential for maintaining bone density, improving posture, and boosting metabolism. If you enjoy feeling strong and challenging yourself, incorporating strength training into your routine is a great choice.

3. **Yoga and Pilates**: Yoga and Pilates focus on flexibility, balance, and core strength. These workouts are excellent for improving posture, reducing stress, and enhancing body awareness. If you prefer a more mindful and gentle approach to exercise, yoga and Pilates can be a wonderful addition to your routine.

4. **HIIT (High-Intensity Interval Training)**: HIIT workouts involve short bursts of intense exercise followed by periods of rest. These workouts are time-efficient and effective for burning calories, improving cardiovascular fitness, and boosting metabolism. If you have limited time but still want to get a challenging workout, HIIT may be the perfect fit for you.

5. **Group Fitness Classes**: Group fitness classes, such as Zumba, kickboxing, or spin classes, offer a fun and social way to exercise. These classes are led by instructors who guide you through a structured workout, making it easier to stay motivated and accountable. If you enjoy the energy and camaraderie of a group setting, joining a fitness class can be a great choice.

Consider Your Schedule and Lifestyle

As a busy working woman, your schedule and lifestyle play a significant role in determining the right workout for you. Consider the following factors:

1. **Time**: How much time can you realistically dedicate to exercise each day or week? If you have limited time, choosing workouts that are shorter but still effective, such as HIIT or circuit training, can be a smart choice.

2. **Location**: Do you prefer working out at home, in a gym, or outdoors? Consider your preferences and the resources available to you. If you enjoy the convenience of working out at home, exploring home workout programs or online fitness classes may be the best option. If you prefer the gym environment or outdoor activities, find a gym or outdoor space that suits your needs.

3. **Flexibility**: Does your schedule vary from day to day or week to week? If so, choosing workouts that offer flexibility, such as online classes or workout apps, can be beneficial. These options allow you to exercise whenever and wherever it fits into your schedule.

4. **Enjoyment**: Ultimately, the key to sticking with a workout routine is finding something you enjoy. If you dread a particular type of exercise, it will be challenging to maintain consistency. Experiment with different workouts until you find something that brings you joy and makes you excited to exercise.

Seek Professional Guidance

If you're unsure about which workout is best for you or how to get started, seeking professional guidance can be incredibly helpful. Consider consulting with a personal trainer, fitness coach, or exercise physiologist who can assess your goals, fitness level, and any specific considerations you may have. They can provide personalized recommendations and create a workout plan tailored to your needs.

Remember, choosing the right workout for you is a personal decision. It's essential to listen to your body, be open to trying new things, and make adjustments along the way. By finding a workout routine that aligns with your goals, preferences, and lifestyle, you can create a sustainable and enjoyable fitness journey.

5.2 Effective Home Workouts

In today's fast-paced world, finding time to exercise can be a challenge, especially for busy working women. Between work commitments, household chores, and family responsibilities, it can feel like there are not enough hours in the day to fit in a workout. However, with the right strategies and a little creativity, you can effectively exercise in the comfort of your own home.

Home workouts offer numerous benefits for the working woman. They provide convenience, flexibility, and privacy, allowing you to exercise on your own terms and at your own pace. Additionally, home workouts eliminate the need for commuting to the gym, saving you valuable time and money. Whether you have a fully equipped home gym or just a small space in your living room, there are plenty of effective exercises you can do to stay fit and healthy.

Designing Your Home Workout Space

Before you start your home workout routine, it's important to create a designated space that is conducive to exercise. This space should be free from distractions and have enough room for you to move comfortably. Clear out any clutter and ensure that you have proper ventilation and lighting. If possible, invest in some basic exercise equipment such as dumbbells, resistance bands, and a yoga mat to enhance your workouts.

Bodyweight Exercises

One of the most effective ways to exercise at home is by incorporating bodyweight exercises into your routine. Bodyweight exercises use your own body as resistance, making them accessible and convenient. They can be modified to suit your fitness level and can target multiple muscle groups at once. Some popular bodyweight exercises include push-ups, squats, lunges, planks, and burpees.

To create a well-rounded workout, choose a variety of bodyweight exercises that target different muscle groups. Aim for a combination of upper body, lower body, and core exercises to ensure a balanced workout. Perform each exercise for a set number of repetitions or for a specific amount of time, depending on your fitness level and goals. As you progress, you can increase the intensity by adding more repetitions or incorporating variations of the exercises.

HIIT Workouts

High-Intensity Interval Training (HIIT) is a popular and effective workout method that can be easily done at home. HIIT workouts involve short bursts of intense exercise followed by brief periods of rest or active recovery. This type of workout is known for its ability to burn calories, improve cardiovascular fitness, and boost metabolism.

To create a HIIT workout at home, choose a combination of exercises that get your heart rate up and challenge your muscles. For example, you can alternate between exercises like jumping jacks, mountain climbers, squat jumps, and high knees. Perform each exercise at maximum effort for a set amount of time, such as 30 seconds, followed by a short rest period of 10-15 seconds. Repeat the circuit for a total of 3-4 rounds.

Online Workout Classes and Apps

If you prefer guidance and structure in your workouts, there are plenty of online workout classes and fitness apps available that cater specifically to home workouts. These resources offer a wide range of workout options, from yoga and Pilates to strength training and cardio. Many of them provide pre-recorded videos or live classes that you can follow along with at your own convenience.

When choosing an online workout class or app, consider your fitness level, goals, and preferences. Look for programs that offer a variety of workouts, clear instructions, and modifications for different fitness levels. Some platforms even provide personalized workout plans and progress tracking features to help you stay motivated and accountable.

Incorporating Cardiovascular Exercise

Cardiovascular exercise is an essential component of any fitness routine, as it helps improve heart health, burn calories, and increase endurance. While traditional cardio exercises like running or cycling may require outdoor space or equipment, there are plenty of ways to get your heart rate up at home.

Jumping rope, dancing, jogging in place, or doing high knees are all effective cardio exercises that can be done in a small space. You can also try following along with cardio workout videos or invest in a compact cardio machine like a stationary bike or elliptical trainer. Aim for at least 150 minutes of moderate-intensity cardio exercise per week, or 75 minutes of vigorous-intensity exercise, spread out over several days.

Creating a Home Workout Routine

To make the most of your home workouts, it's important to establish a consistent routine. Set aside dedicated time each day or week for exercise and treat it as a non-negotiable appointment with yourself. Consider your schedule and energy levels when planning your workouts, and be realistic about the time and effort you can commit.

Start by setting specific goals for your home workouts. Whether you want to improve strength, increase flexibility, or lose weight, having clear goals will help you stay focused and motivated. Break down your goals into smaller, achievable milestones and track your progress along the way. Celebrate your successes and adjust your routine as needed to keep challenging yourself.

Remember to warm up before each workout and cool down afterward to prevent injury and promote recovery. Stretching exercises, such as yoga or Pilates, can also be incorporated into your routine to improve flexibility and promote relaxation.

Conclusion

Effective home workouts are a valuable tool for busy working women who want to prioritize their fitness and well-being. By creating a designated workout space, incorporating bodyweight exercises and HIIT workouts, utilizing online resources, and incorporating cardiovascular exercise, you can achieve your fitness goals from the comfort of your own home. With consistency, dedication, and a positive mindset, you can maintain a healthy and balanced lifestyle while juggling the demands of work and family.

5.3 Maximizing Gym Sessions

When it comes to maximizing your gym sessions, preparation and planning are key. As a busy working woman, your time is valuable, so making the most of your workouts is essential. In this section, we will explore strategies and tips to help you optimize your gym sessions and achieve your fitness goals.

1. Set Clear Goals

Before heading to the gym, it's important to have a clear understanding of what you want to achieve. Whether your goal is to lose weight, build strength, or improve your overall fitness, having a specific objective will help you stay focused and motivated during your workouts. Take some time to write down your goals and break them down into smaller, achievable targets. This will give you a sense of direction and purpose when you step into the gym.

2. Plan Your Workouts

To make the most of your gym sessions, it's crucial to have a well-structured workout plan. This plan should include a variety of exercises that target different muscle groups and incorporate both cardiovascular and strength training. Consider seeking guidance from a personal trainer or fitness professional to help you design a customized workout plan that aligns with your goals and fitness level. Having a plan in place will not only save you time but also ensure that you are making progress towards your goals.

3. Warm Up Properly

Before diving into your workout, it's essential to warm up your body to prevent injuries and prepare your muscles for the upcoming exercises. Spend at least 5-10 minutes engaging in dynamic stretches and light cardio activities such as jogging or cycling. This will increase your heart rate, improve blood flow to your muscles, and enhance your overall performance during the workout.

4. Focus on Compound Exercises

Compound exercises are multi-joint movements that engage multiple muscle groups simultaneously. These exercises are highly effective for maximizing your gym sessions as they allow you to work multiple muscles in a shorter amount of time. Examples of compound exercises include squats, deadlifts, lunges, bench presses, and pull-ups. Incorporating these exercises into your routine will help you build strength, burn calories, and improve your overall fitness level.

5. Incorporate High-Intensity Interval Training (HIIT)

If you're short on time but still want to get an effective workout, consider incorporating high-intensity interval training (HIIT) into your gym sessions. HIIT involves alternating between short bursts of intense exercise and brief recovery periods. This type of training has been shown to be highly efficient in burning calories, improving cardiovascular fitness, and boosting metabolism. You can incorporate HIIT into your gym sessions by adding intervals of intense cardio exercises such as sprints, burpees, or jump squats.

6. Use Supersets and Circuit Training

To maximize your time at the gym, consider incorporating supersets and circuit training into your workouts. Supersets involve performing two exercises back-to-back without resting in between. This allows you to work different muscle groups consecutively, saving you time and increasing the intensity of your workout. Circuit training involves performing a series of exercises one after another with minimal rest in between. This method keeps your heart rate elevated and targets multiple muscle groups, providing a full-body workout in a shorter amount of time.

7. Track Your Progress

Tracking your progress is essential for staying motivated and ensuring that you are making progress towards your goals. Keep a workout journal or use a fitness tracking app to record your exercises, sets, reps, and weights. This will help you monitor your progress, identify areas for improvement, and make adjustments to your workout plan as needed. Additionally, seeing your progress on paper can be incredibly motivating and serve as a reminder of how far you've come.

8. Stay Hydrated and Fuel Your Body

Proper hydration and nutrition are crucial for maximizing your gym sessions. Make sure to drink plenty of water before, during, and after your workouts to stay hydrated. Additionally, fuel your body with a balanced meal or snack containing carbohydrates and protein before your gym session. This will provide you with the energy you need to perform at your best and aid in muscle recovery.

9. Listen to Your Body

While pushing yourself during workouts is important, it's equally important to listen to your body and avoid overtraining or pushing beyond your limits. Pay attention to any signs of fatigue, pain, or discomfort and adjust your workout intensity or take rest days as needed. Remember, rest and recovery are just as important as the actual workout in achieving optimal results.

10. Make the Most of Your Time

As a busy working woman, time is often limited. To make the most of your gym sessions, minimize distractions and stay focused on your workout. Put your phone on silent or airplane mode to avoid interruptions and distractions. Use your rest periods effectively by stretching or performing active recovery exercises instead of scrolling through social media. By staying focused and making the most of your time at the gym, you'll be able to achieve more in less time.

Remember, consistency is key when it comes to maximizing your gym sessions. Aim to make exercise a regular part of your routine and prioritize your workouts just like any other important commitment in your life. With proper planning, focus, and dedication, you can make the most of your gym sessions and achieve your fitness goals while balancing your work and personal life.

5.4 Incorporating Cardiovascular Exercise

Cardiovascular exercise, also known as cardio or aerobic exercise, is an essential component of any fitness routine. It helps improve heart health, increase stamina, burn calories, and boost overall fitness levels. For busy women, finding time to incorporate cardiovascular exercise into their daily lives can be a challenge. However, with some strategic planning and creative thinking, it is possible to make cardio workouts a regular part of your routine. In this section, we will explore various ways to incorporate cardiovascular exercise into your busy schedule.

1. Prioritize Your Cardiovascular Health

Before we dive into the strategies, it's important to understand the significance of cardiovascular exercise for your overall health. Regular cardio workouts can help reduce the risk of heart disease, lower blood pressure, improve cholesterol levels, and enhance lung function. By prioritizing your cardiovascular health, you are investing in a healthier and more energetic future.

2. Choose Activities You Enjoy

The key to sticking with any exercise routine is to choose activities that you genuinely enjoy. If you dread your cardio workouts, it will be challenging to stay motivated and consistent. Consider trying different activities such as running, cycling, swimming, dancing, kickboxing, or even brisk walking. Experiment with different options until you find something that excites you and keeps you engaged.

3. Make the Most of Your Commute

For many working women, commuting to and from work takes up a significant portion of their day. Instead of sitting in traffic or on public transportation, consider alternative modes of transportation that allow you to incorporate cardiovascular exercise. If possible, try walking or biking to work. Not only will this help you get your cardio in, but it will also save you money on transportation costs and reduce your carbon footprint.

4. Utilize Your Lunch Break

Instead of spending your entire lunch break sitting at your desk or in the break room, use this time to squeeze in a quick cardio workout. You can go for a brisk walk or jog around your office building or find a nearby park to get some fresh air. If you have access to a gym or fitness center, consider using this time to hop on a treadmill, stationary bike, or elliptical machine. Even just 20-30 minutes of cardio during your lunch break can make a significant difference in your overall fitness.

5. Incorporate Cardio into Household Chores

As a busy woman, you likely have a never-ending to-do list when it comes to household chores. Instead of viewing these tasks as a burden, think of them as an opportunity to get your heart rate up. Activities like vacuuming, mopping, gardening, or even cleaning the windows can be surprisingly effective at getting your blood pumping. Put on some energetic music and turn your chores into a cardio workout.

6. Schedule Active Breaks

If you have a sedentary job that requires long hours of sitting, it's crucial to incorporate regular active breaks into your workday. Set a timer to remind yourself to get up and move every hour. Use these breaks to do a quick cardio routine, such as jumping jacks, high knees, or marching in place. Not only will this help you stay active, but it will also boost your energy levels and improve your focus.

7. Join Group Fitness Classes

Group fitness classes are a fantastic way to incorporate cardiovascular exercise into your routine while also enjoying the social aspect of working out. Look for classes that focus on cardio-intensive activities like Zumba, spinning, kickboxing, or dance aerobics. Not only will you get a great workout, but you'll also have the opportunity to meet like-minded individuals who can provide support and motivation.

8. Make Family Time Active

If you have a family, finding time for exercise can be even more challenging. However, you can turn family time into an opportunity for cardiovascular exercise. Instead of spending your weekends sitting on the couch watching movies, plan active outings such as hiking, biking, or playing a game of soccer in the park. Not only will you be spending quality time with your loved ones, but you'll also be setting a positive example of an active and healthy lifestyle.

9. Set Realistic Goals

When incorporating cardiovascular exercise into your busy schedule, it's essential to set realistic goals. Start by committing to a certain number of cardio sessions per week and gradually increase the duration and intensity as you progress. Remember, consistency is key, so even if you can only fit in short workouts initially, it's better than not doing anything at all. Celebrate your small victories and keep pushing yourself to reach new milestones.

10. Stay Flexible and Adapt

Life is unpredictable, and there will be times when your schedule gets disrupted. It's important to stay flexible and adapt your cardio routine accordingly. If you can't make it to the gym, find alternative ways to get your heart rate up, such as following an online workout video or going for a run in your neighborhood. The key is to find solutions rather than making excuses.

Incorporating cardiovascular exercise into your busy life as a working woman may require some creativity and planning, but it is entirely possible. By prioritizing your cardiovascular health, choosing activities you enjoy, and making the most of your available time, you can achieve a balanced and active lifestyle. Remember, every step counts, so start small and build momentum as you go.

Strength Training for Women

6.1 Understanding the Benefits of Strength Training

Strength training is a crucial component of any fitness routine, especially for women. It involves using resistance to build and strengthen muscles, resulting in numerous physical and mental benefits. In this section, we will explore the various advantages of incorporating strength training into your workout regimen.

Building Lean Muscle Mass

One of the primary benefits of strength training is the ability to build lean muscle mass. Contrary to popular belief, strength training will not make you bulky or masculine. Instead, it helps you develop a toned and sculpted physique. As women age, they naturally lose muscle mass, which can lead to a decrease in metabolism and an increase in body fat. By engaging in regular strength training, you can counteract this process and maintain a healthy body composition.

Boosting Metabolism

Strength training has a significant impact on your metabolism. Unlike cardio exercises that primarily burn calories during the workout, strength training increases your metabolic rate even after you've finished exercising. This is because building and maintaining muscle requires more energy than fat. By incorporating strength training into your routine, you can elevate your resting metabolic rate, allowing you to burn more calories throughout the day, even when you're at rest.

Enhancing Bone Health

Osteoporosis, a condition characterized by weak and brittle bones, is more prevalent in women than men. Strength training plays a vital role in maintaining and improving bone health. When you engage in weight-bearing exercises, such as lifting weights or using resistance bands, you stimulate bone growth and increase bone density. This can help prevent osteoporosis and reduce the risk of fractures and injuries as you age.

Improving Functional Strength and Balance

Strength training not only helps you look and feel stronger but also improves your functional strength and balance. As a working woman, you need to be able to perform daily tasks with ease and confidence. By strengthening your muscles, you enhance your ability to lift and carry heavy objects, climb stairs, and perform other physical activities required in your daily life. Additionally, strength training can improve your balance and stability, reducing the risk of falls and injuries.

Enhancing Posture and Joint Stability

Sitting at a desk for long hours or engaging in repetitive movements can lead to poor posture and joint instability. Strength training can help correct these issues by strengthening the muscles that support your spine and joints. By improving your posture, you can alleviate back and neck pain, reduce the risk of injuries, and enhance your overall physical appearance.

Boosting Confidence and Mental Well-being

Strength training not only has physical benefits but also has a positive impact on your mental well-being. As you become stronger and more capable, you gain confidence in your abilities. This newfound confidence can extend beyond the gym and positively impact other areas of your life, including your career. Additionally, strength training releases endorphins, which are natural mood boosters. Regular exercise can help reduce stress, anxiety, and symptoms of depression, leaving you feeling more energized and mentally resilient.

Preventing Chronic Diseases

Engaging in regular strength training can significantly reduce the risk of chronic diseases such as heart disease, diabetes, and certain types of cancer. Strength training improves insulin sensitivity, which helps regulate blood sugar levels and reduces the risk of developing type 2 diabetes. It also helps lower blood pressure and cholesterol levels, reducing the risk of heart disease. Additionally, strength training has been shown to decrease the risk of certain types of cancer, including breast and colon cancer.

Empowering Independence and Longevity

As a working woman, it's essential to maintain your independence and enjoy a high quality of life as you age. Strength training can help you achieve this by improving your physical capabilities and overall health. By building strength and maintaining muscle mass, you can continue to perform daily activities independently and reduce the risk of age-related health issues. Strength training is a powerful tool that empowers you to live a long, active, and fulfilling life.

Incorporating strength training into your fitness routine is essential for achieving optimal health and well-being. It offers a wide range of benefits, from building lean muscle mass and boosting metabolism to improving bone health and enhancing mental well-being. By understanding and harnessing the power of strength training, you can take control of your physical and mental health, allowing you to thrive both personally and professionally.

6.2 Designing a Strength Training Program

Strength training is a crucial component of any fitness routine, especially for women. It not only helps build lean muscle mass but also improves bone density, boosts metabolism, and enhances overall strength and functionality. Designing a well-rounded strength training program is essential to maximize the benefits and achieve your fitness goals. In this section, we will explore the key elements of designing an effective strength training program specifically tailored for busy women.

Understanding Your Goals

Before diving into designing a strength training program, it's important to identify your specific goals. Are you looking to build muscle, increase strength, improve overall fitness, or enhance athletic performance? Understanding your goals will help you tailor your program to meet your individual needs.

Assessing Your Current Fitness Level

To design an effective strength training program, it's crucial to assess your current fitness level. This will help you determine the appropriate starting point and progress at a safe and manageable pace. Consider factors such as your current strength, endurance, flexibility, and any existing injuries or limitations. If you're unsure about your fitness level, consulting with a qualified fitness professional can provide valuable insights and guidance.

Choosing the Right Exercises

When designing a strength training program, it's important to include a variety of exercises that target different muscle groups. Compound exercises, which involve multiple muscle groups, are particularly effective for maximizing strength gains and overall muscle development. Some examples of compound exercises include squats, deadlifts, lunges, bench presses, and rows.

In addition to compound exercises, it's also beneficial to include isolation exercises that target specific muscle groups. These exercises can help address any muscle imbalances and provide additional focus on areas you want to develop further. Examples of isolation exercises include bicep curls, tricep extensions, calf raises, and lateral raises.

Determining Sets, Reps, and Rest Periods

To effectively stimulate muscle growth and strength gains, it's important to determine the appropriate number of sets, reps, and rest periods for each exercise. The number of sets and reps will depend on your goals and fitness level. Generally, performing 2-4 sets of 8-12 reps per exercise is a good starting point for building strength and muscle endurance.

Rest periods between sets are also crucial for recovery and optimal performance. Shorter rest periods (30-60 seconds) are typically recommended for improving muscular endurance, while longer rest periods (1-3 minutes) are more suitable for maximizing strength gains. Adjusting rest periods based on your goals and fitness level can help optimize your training sessions.

Progression and Periodization

To continue making progress and avoid plateaus, it's important to incorporate progression and periodization into your strength training program. Progression involves gradually increasing the intensity, volume, or complexity of your workouts over time. This can be achieved by increasing the weight, adding more reps or sets, or incorporating more challenging variations of exercises.

Periodization involves dividing your training program into specific phases or cycles, each with a different focus or goal. This allows for structured variation and prevents overtraining or stagnation. Common periodization models include linear periodization, where intensity and volume gradually increase over time, and undulating periodization, which involves alternating between different training variables within each week or training cycle.

Balancing Strength Training with Other Forms of Exercise

While strength training is essential, it's important to balance it with other forms of exercise to maintain overall fitness and prevent overuse injuries. Incorporating cardiovascular exercise, such as running, cycling, or swimming, can help improve cardiovascular health and burn additional calories. Flexibility and mobility exercises, such as yoga or Pilates, can enhance joint range of motion and prevent muscle imbalances.

Listening to Your Body

Lastly, it's crucial to listen to your body and make adjustments as needed. Pay attention to any signs of fatigue, pain, or discomfort during your workouts. If something doesn't feel right, it's important to modify or seek guidance from a qualified professional. Rest and recovery are just as important as training, so make sure to prioritize adequate rest days and listen to your body's signals.

Designing a strength training program that suits your goals, fitness level, and lifestyle is key to achieving long-term success. By incorporating a variety of exercises, determining appropriate sets and reps, and incorporating progression and periodization, you can create a program that challenges you and helps you reach your full potential. Remember to always prioritize safety, listen to your body, and enjoy the journey of becoming stronger and more empowered through strength training.

6.3 Proper Form and Technique

When it comes to strength training, proper form and technique are essential for maximizing results and preventing injuries. Whether you're a beginner or an experienced lifter, understanding and practicing correct form is crucial for getting the most out of your workouts. In this section, we will explore the importance of proper form and technique in strength training and provide you with some tips to ensure you're performing exercises correctly.

Why Proper Form Matters

Performing exercises with proper form is essential for several reasons. First and foremost, it helps to target the intended muscles effectively. When you use correct form, you engage the specific muscles you're trying to work, allowing for optimal muscle activation and growth. On the other hand, using improper form can lead to compensations and imbalances, which may result in muscle imbalances and potential injuries.

Secondly, proper form ensures that you're using the correct muscles throughout the movement. It's common for individuals to rely on momentum or other muscle groups to complete an exercise, rather than the targeted muscles. This not only diminishes the effectiveness of the exercise but also increases the risk of injury.

Lastly, maintaining proper form helps to improve your overall body mechanics and posture. Many strength training exercises require core stability and proper alignment, which can translate into better posture and reduced risk of back pain or other postural issues.

Tips for Proper Form and Technique

Now that we understand the importance of proper form, let's dive into some tips to help you maintain correct technique during your strength training sessions:

1. Start with a Warm-up Before diving into your strength training routine, it's crucial to warm up your muscles and joints. A proper warm-up increases blood flow to the muscles, improves flexibility, and prepares your body for the upcoming workout. Incorporate dynamic stretches and light cardio exercises to warm up your entire body.

2. Focus on Alignment Proper alignment is key to maintaining good form during strength training exercises. Pay attention to your posture and ensure that your spine is neutral, shoulders are relaxed, and core is engaged. Avoid rounding your back or hunching your shoulders, as this can put unnecessary strain on your spine and increase the risk of injury.

3. Control the Movement One common mistake people make during strength training is using momentum to complete the exercise. Instead, focus on controlling the movement throughout the entire range of motion. This ensures that you're engaging the targeted muscles fully and reduces the risk of relying on other muscle groups to compensate.

4. Engage the Core Your core plays a crucial role in maintaining stability and proper form during strength training exercises. Before starting any movement, engage your core by drawing your belly button towards your spine. This helps to stabilize your spine and protect your lower back.

5. Breathe Properly Proper breathing technique is often overlooked but is essential for maintaining proper form and maximizing performance. Inhale during the eccentric (lowering) phase of the exercise and exhale during the concentric (lifting) phase. This helps to stabilize your core and maintain proper intra-abdominal pressure.

6. Start with Light Weights If you're new to strength training or trying out a new exercise, it's best to start with lighter weights. This allows you to focus on your form and technique without compromising your safety. As you become more comfortable and confident, gradually increase the weight while maintaining proper form.

7. Use a Mirror or Record Yourself Using a mirror or recording yourself while performing exercises can be a helpful tool for assessing your form. It allows you to visually observe your movements and make any necessary adjustments. Pay attention to your body positioning, joint alignment, and range of motion.

8. Seek Professional Guidance If you're unsure about proper form or technique, consider seeking guidance from a qualified fitness professional. They can provide personalized instruction, correct any form errors, and ensure that you're performing exercises safely and effectively.

Common Form Mistakes to Avoid

While it's important to focus on proper form, it's equally crucial to be aware of common form mistakes and avoid them. Here are a few common form mistakes to watch out for:

1. Rounded Back Rounding your back during exercises such as deadlifts or rows can put excessive stress on your spine and increase the risk of injury. Focus on maintaining a neutral spine throughout the movement.

2. Overarching Lower Back Hyperextending or overarching your lower back, especially during exercises like squats or overhead presses, can strain your lower back and lead to discomfort or injury. Engage your core and maintain a slight natural curve in your lower back.

3. Lifting Shoulders during Upper Body Exercises When performing upper body exercises like shoulder presses or bicep curls, avoid shrugging your shoulders. Keep your shoulders relaxed and down, away from your ears, to prevent unnecessary tension in your neck and shoulders.

4. Using Momentum Swinging or using momentum to lift weights takes away the focus from the targeted muscles and increases the risk of injury. Instead, focus on controlled movements and avoid relying on momentum to complete the exercise.

5. Neglecting Full Range of Motion Performing exercises with a limited range of motion can limit the benefits and effectiveness of the exercise. Aim to complete the full range of motion while maintaining proper form and control throughout.

By focusing on proper form and technique, you can make the most out of your strength training workouts while minimizing the risk of injuries. Remember to start with lighter weights, seek professional guidance if needed, and always prioritize safety and proper alignment. With consistent practice and attention to form, you'll be well on your way to achieving your fitness goals.

6.4 Progression and Overcoming Plateaus

As you continue on your strength training journey, it's important to understand the concept of progression and how to overcome plateaus. Progression refers to the gradual increase in the intensity, duration, or complexity of your workouts over time. It is a key factor in achieving continuous improvement and avoiding stagnation in your fitness journey. Plateaus, on the other hand, are periods where you may feel stuck or not see any further progress despite your efforts. In this section, we will explore strategies to help you progress in your strength training and overcome plateaus.

Understanding Progression

Progression is essential for building strength and muscle. When you consistently challenge your body with increased demands, it adapts by becoming stronger and more efficient. There are several ways to progress in your strength training routine:

1. **Increasing Resistance**: One of the most common ways to progress is by gradually increasing the weight or resistance you use during your exercises. This can be done by adding more weight to your dumbbells, using resistance bands with higher tension, or using weight machines with heavier settings.

2. **Increasing Repetitions**: Another way to progress is by gradually increasing the number of repetitions you perform for each exercise. As your muscles become stronger, you can gradually add more repetitions to your sets. This helps to further challenge your muscles and stimulate growth.

3. **Increasing Sets**: Increasing the number of sets you perform for each exercise is another way to progress. Adding an extra set can increase the overall volume of your workout, providing a greater stimulus for muscle growth.

4. **Decreasing Rest Time**: Reducing the amount of rest time between sets can also be a form of progression. By shortening your rest periods, you increase the intensity of your workout and challenge your muscles to work harder.

5. **Changing Exercise Variations**: Introducing new exercise variations or variations that target different muscle groups can also be a form of progression. This helps to prevent your body from adapting to the same exercises and stimulates new muscle growth.

Overcoming Plateaus

Plateaus are a common occurrence in any fitness journey. They can be frustrating and demotivating, but they are also an opportunity for growth and learning. Here are some strategies to help you overcome plateaus and continue making progress:

1. **Evaluate Your Routine**: Take a step back and evaluate your current strength training routine. Are you consistently challenging yourself? Are you using proper form and technique? Are you incorporating enough variety in your exercises? Sometimes, making small adjustments to your routine can make a big difference in breaking through plateaus.

2. **Increase Intensity**: If you've been using the same weight or resistance for a while, it may be time to increase the intensity. Gradually increase the weight or resistance you use for your exercises to provide a greater challenge for your muscles.

3. **Try Different Training Methods**: Incorporating different training methods can help you overcome plateaus. For example, if you've been primarily using free weights, try incorporating resistance machines or

bodyweight exercises into your routine. This change in stimulus can help kickstart progress.

4. **Focus on Weak Areas**: Identify any weak areas or muscle imbalances in your body and target them specifically. By focusing on these areas, you can improve overall strength and address any imbalances that may be hindering your progress.

5. **Periodize Your Training**: Periodization involves dividing your training into different phases, each with a specific focus and intensity level. By incorporating periodization into your strength training routine, you can prevent plateaus and continue making progress.

6. **Rest and Recovery**: Sometimes, plateaus can be a sign that your body needs rest and recovery. Make sure you are allowing enough time for rest days and prioritizing sleep. Proper rest and recovery are crucial for muscle growth and overall performance.

7. **Seek Professional Guidance**: If you're struggling to overcome a plateau, consider seeking guidance from a fitness professional. They can assess your current routine, provide personalized recommendations, and help you break through the plateau.

Remember, plateaus are a normal part of the fitness journey. Embrace them as an opportunity to learn and grow. By implementing these strategies and staying consistent, you can overcome plateaus and continue progressing in your strength training journey.

Keep pushing yourself, stay motivated, and celebrate your achievements along the way. Your dedication and hard work will pay off, and you will continue to see improvements in your strength, fitness, and overall well-being.

Flexibility and Mobility

7.1 The Importance of Flexibility and Mobility

Flexibility and mobility are often overlooked aspects of fitness, but they play a crucial role in maintaining overall health and well-being. In this section, we will explore why flexibility and mobility are important for working women and how they can enhance your physical performance and prevent injuries.

The Benefits of Flexibility

Flexibility refers to the ability of your muscles and joints to move through their full range of motion. It is an essential component of fitness that can bring numerous benefits to your body and mind. Here are some key advantages of incorporating flexibility exercises into your fitness routine:

1. **Improved posture**: Flexibility exercises help lengthen tight muscles and release tension, which can improve your posture and reduce the risk of developing musculoskeletal imbalances.

2. **Enhanced athletic performance**: Increased flexibility allows for greater joint mobility, which can improve your performance in various physical activities, such as running, weightlifting, and yoga.

3. **Injury prevention**: Flexible muscles and joints are less prone to injuries, as they can better absorb impact and adapt to sudden movements or changes in direction.

4. **Reduced muscle soreness**: Regular stretching after exercise can help alleviate muscle soreness and promote faster recovery.

5. **Stress relief**: Flexibility exercises, such as yoga or stretching, can help relax both your body and mind, reducing stress and promoting a sense of calm.

The Importance of Mobility

While flexibility focuses on the range of motion of your muscles and joints, mobility encompasses the ability to move freely and efficiently in different planes of motion. Mobility exercises target not only the muscles but also the surrounding connective tissues, ligaments, and tendons. Here's why mobility is crucial for working women:

1. **Functional movement**: Mobility exercises improve your ability to perform everyday tasks, such as bending, lifting, and reaching, with ease and without pain or discomfort.

2. **Joint health**: Maintaining good joint mobility helps prevent stiffness, reduces the risk of joint degeneration, and promotes overall joint health.

3. **Balance and stability**: Mobility exercises challenge your body's balance and stability, improving your coordination and reducing the risk of falls or accidents.

4. **Enhanced performance**: By improving your mobility, you can optimize your movement patterns and enhance your performance in various physical activities, including sports and exercise routines.

5. **Injury prevention**: Adequate mobility reduces the risk of muscle imbalances and compensatory movements, which can lead to overuse injuries or chronic pain.

Incorporating Flexibility and Mobility Exercises

Now that you understand the importance of flexibility and mobility, it's time to incorporate specific exercises into your fitness routine. Here are some effective ways to improve your flexibility and mobility:

1. **Dynamic warm-up**: Before engaging in any physical activity, start with a dynamic warm-up routine that includes movements that mimic the activity you're about to perform. This helps prepare your muscles and joints for the upcoming workout.

2. **Static stretching**: After your workout or on rest days, perform static stretches that target major muscle groups. Hold each stretch for 15-30 seconds and repeat 2-3 times. Focus on areas that feel tight or restricted.

3. **Yoga and Pilates**: Consider adding yoga or Pilates classes to your fitness routine. These practices not only improve flexibility and mobility but also promote relaxation and stress reduction.

4. **Foam rolling and self-myofascial release**: Use a foam roller or other self-massage tools to release tension in your muscles and fascia. Roll slowly over tight areas, pausing on any tender spots for 20-30 seconds.

5. **Incorporate mobility exercises**: Include exercises that target specific joints and movement patterns, such as hip openers, shoulder mobility drills, and spinal twists. These exercises can be done as part of your warm-up or as standalone sessions.

Remember to listen to your body and progress gradually. Flexibility and mobility take time to improve, so be patient and consistent with your practice. As a working woman, it's essential to prioritize your physical well-being and make time for these exercises to reap the benefits they offer.

In conclusion, flexibility and mobility are vital components of a well-rounded fitness routine for working women. They improve posture, enhance athletic performance, prevent injuries, reduce muscle soreness, and promote stress relief. By incorporating flexibility and mobility exercises into your routine, you can optimize your movement patterns, improve joint health, and enhance your overall physical performance. So, make it a priority to stretch, move, and take care of your body to achieve a balanced and healthy lifestyle.

7.2 Stretching and Warm-up Exercises

Stretching and warm-up exercises are essential components of any fitness routine, especially for busy women who are constantly juggling work and other responsibilities. These exercises not only help prevent injuries but also improve flexibility, enhance performance, and promote overall well-being. In this section, we will explore the importance of stretching and warm-up exercises and provide you with a variety of exercises that you can easily incorporate into your daily routine.

The Importance of Stretching and Warm-up Exercises

Before diving into the specific exercises, let's first understand why stretching and warm-up exercises are crucial for your fitness journey. Here are some key benefits:

1. **Injury Prevention:** Stretching and warming up your muscles before exercise helps increase blood flow, oxygen delivery, and nutrient supply to the muscles. This prepares your body for physical activity and reduces the risk of muscle strains, sprains, and other injuries.

2. **Improved Flexibility:** Regular stretching can improve your flexibility and range of motion. This is particularly important for women who spend long hours sitting at a desk or engaging in repetitive movements. Stretching helps counteract the negative effects of prolonged sitting and promotes better posture.

3. **Enhanced Performance:** When you warm up your body before a workout, you increase your heart rate, body temperature, and blood flow to the muscles. This primes your body for physical activity, improves muscle contraction, and enhances overall performance during your workout.

4. **Reduced Muscle Soreness:** Stretching after a workout can help reduce muscle soreness and stiffness. It aids in the removal of waste products, such as lactic acid, from the muscles, which can accumulate during exercise and contribute to post-workout discomfort.

5. **Stress Relief:** Stretching and warm-up exercises can also have a positive impact on your mental well-being. They promote relaxation, reduce stress levels, and provide an opportunity for mindfulness and self-care.

Stretching Exercises

Now that you understand the importance of stretching and warm-up exercises, let's explore some specific stretches that you can incorporate into your routine. Remember to perform these exercises in a controlled manner, without bouncing or jerking movements, and hold each stretch for 15-30 seconds.

1. **Neck Stretch:** Gently tilt your head to one side, bringing your ear towards your shoulder. Hold for 15-30 seconds and repeat on the other side. This stretch helps relieve tension in the neck and upper back.

2. **Shoulder Stretch:** Extend one arm across your chest and use the opposite hand to gently pull the arm closer to your body. Hold for 15-30 seconds and repeat on the other side. This stretch targets the muscles in your shoulders and upper back.

3. **Chest Opener:** Stand tall with your feet hip-width apart. Interlace your fingers behind your back and gently lift your arms away from your body, keeping your chest open. Hold for 15-30 seconds. This stretch helps counteract the forward rounding of the shoulders caused by prolonged sitting.

4. **Hamstring Stretch:** Sit on the edge of a chair with one leg extended in

front of you. Keeping your back straight, hinge forward from your hips until you feel a gentle stretch in the back of your thigh. Hold for 15-30 seconds and repeat on the other leg. This stretch targets the hamstrings.

5. **Quadriceps Stretch:** Stand tall and hold onto a wall or chair for support if needed. Bend one knee and bring your heel towards your glutes, grabbing your ankle or foot with your hand. Hold for 15-30 seconds and repeat on the other leg. This stretch targets the front of your thigh.

Warm-up Exercises

In addition to stretching, incorporating warm-up exercises into your routine is equally important. Warm-up exercises gradually increase your heart rate, body temperature, and blood flow to the muscles, preparing your body for more intense physical activity. Here are some effective warm-up exercises:

1. **Marching in Place:** Stand tall and march in place, lifting your knees as high as comfortable. Continue for 1-2 minutes to gradually increase your heart rate and warm up your leg muscles.

2. **Arm Circles:** Stand with your feet shoulder-width apart and extend your arms out to the sides. Make small circles with your arms, gradually increasing the size of the circles. After 15-30 seconds, reverse the direction of the circles. This exercise warms up your shoulder joints and upper body.

3. **Jumping Jacks:** Start with your feet together and arms by your sides. Jump your feet out to the sides while simultaneously raising your arms overhead. Jump back to the starting position and repeat for 1-2 minutes. Jumping jacks increase your heart rate, warm up your entire body, and improve coordination.

4. **High Knees:** Stand tall and march in place, lifting your knees as high as possible. Aim to bring your knees up to hip level. Continue for 1-2 minutes to warm up your leg muscles and increase your heart rate.

5. **Hip Circles:** Stand with your feet hip-width apart and place your hands on your hips. Make circular motions with your hips, gradually increasing the size of the circles. After 15-30 seconds, reverse the direction of the circles. This exercise warms up your hip joints and lower body.

Remember to listen to your body and modify or skip any exercises that cause pain or discomfort. Incorporating stretching and warm-up exercises into your fitness routine will not only help you prevent injuries but also enhance your overall performance and well-being. So, take a few extra minutes before each workout to prioritize these important exercises. Your body will thank you!

7.3 Yoga and Pilates for Flexibility

Yoga and Pilates are two popular forms of exercise that focus on flexibility, strength, and mindfulness. These practices can be incredibly beneficial for working women who are looking to improve their overall fitness and find balance in their lives. In this section, we will explore the benefits of yoga and Pilates for flexibility and how you can incorporate these practices into your fitness routine.

The Benefits of Yoga for Flexibility

Yoga is a centuries-old practice that combines physical postures, breathing exercises, and meditation. One of the main benefits of yoga is its ability to improve flexibility. Through a series of stretching and lengthening movements, yoga helps to increase the range of motion in your joints and muscles.

Flexibility is essential for maintaining good posture, preventing injuries, and enhancing athletic performance. As a working woman, you may spend long hours sitting at a desk or engaging in repetitive movements. This can lead to tight muscles and limited mobility. Yoga can help counteract these effects by stretching and elongating the muscles, promoting better alignment, and relieving tension in the body.

Additionally, yoga can improve your overall body awareness and proprioception, which is your ability to sense the position of your body in space. This heightened awareness can help you move more efficiently and with greater ease throughout your day.

Incorporating Yoga into Your Fitness Routine

If you're new to yoga, it's best to start with beginner-friendly classes or online tutorials. Many yoga studios offer classes specifically designed for beginners, which focus on foundational poses and proper alignment. These classes are a great way to learn the basics and build a strong yoga practice.

When incorporating yoga into your fitness routine, aim for at least two to three sessions per week. This will allow you to experience the benefits of regular practice and gradually improve your flexibility over time. You can choose to attend in-person classes, follow online videos, or even create your own routine at home.

To get started, set aside a dedicated space in your home where you can practice yoga without distractions. Invest in a yoga mat and any props that may be helpful, such as blocks or straps. Begin each session with a few minutes of deep breathing and gentle stretching to warm up your body.

As you progress, you can explore different styles of yoga, such as Hatha, Vinyasa, or Yin. Each style offers unique benefits and focuses on different aspects of the practice. Experiment with different classes and instructors to find what resonates with you and fits your schedule.

The Benefits of Pilates for Flexibility

Pilates is a low-impact exercise method that focuses on core strength, flexibility, and body awareness. It was developed by Joseph Pilates in the early 20th century and has gained popularity worldwide. While Pilates is known for its core-strengthening benefits, it also plays a significant role in improving flexibility.

Pilates exercises are designed to lengthen and strengthen the muscles, particularly those in the core, back, hips, and legs. By engaging in controlled movements and emphasizing proper alignment, Pilates helps to improve posture and increase flexibility.

One of the unique aspects of Pilates is its focus on the mind-body connection. Each movement is performed with precision and control, requiring concentration and mindfulness. This mindful approach to exercise can help you develop a deeper understanding of your body and its capabilities, leading to improved flexibility and overall physical well-being.

Incorporating Pilates into Your Fitness Routine

Similar to yoga, Pilates can be practiced in a variety of settings, including studios, gyms, or at home. If you're new to Pilates, it's recommended to start with a beginner's class or work with a certified instructor who can guide you through the exercises and ensure proper form.

When incorporating Pilates into your fitness routine, aim for two to three sessions per week. Each session typically lasts around 45 minutes to an hour. You can choose to attend group classes or opt for private sessions if you prefer more personalized instruction.

If you prefer to practice Pilates at home, there are many online resources available, including video tutorials and virtual classes. Invest in a Pilates mat or use a thick exercise mat to provide cushioning and support for your body during the exercises.

When starting a Pilates session, begin with a warm-up that includes gentle stretches and mobilization exercises for the spine. This will prepare your body for the more challenging movements that follow. Throughout the session, focus on maintaining proper alignment and engaging your core muscles to maximize the benefits of each exercise.

As you progress in your Pilates practice, you can incorporate props such as resistance bands, stability balls, or Pilates rings to add variety and challenge to your workouts. These props can help deepen your stretches and increase the intensity of your Pilates sessions.

Conclusion

Yoga and Pilates are excellent practices for improving flexibility, strength, and overall well-being. By incorporating these exercises into your fitness routine, you can enhance your physical performance, reduce the risk of injuries, and find balance in your busy life as a working woman. Whether you choose to attend classes or practice at home, remember to listen to your body, start slowly, and gradually increase the intensity and duration of your sessions. With consistency and dedication, you will experience the transformative benefits of yoga and Pilates for flexibility.

7.4 Foam Rolling and Self-Myofascial Release

Foam rolling and self-myofascial release are essential techniques that can help working women improve their flexibility, mobility, and overall well-being. These practices involve using a foam roller or other tools to apply pressure to specific areas of the body, releasing tension and promoting muscle recovery. In this section, we will explore the benefits of foam rolling, how to incorporate it into your fitness routine, and some key techniques to get you started.

The Benefits of Foam Rolling

Foam rolling offers numerous benefits for working women who are looking to enhance their fitness and overall health. Here are some of the key advantages of incorporating foam rolling into your routine:

1. **Improved Flexibility and Range of Motion**: Foam rolling helps to release tight muscles and fascia, which can improve your flexibility and range of motion. By targeting specific areas of tension, you can increase your body's ability to move freely and perform exercises with proper form.

2. **Enhanced Muscle Recovery**: Foam rolling aids in muscle recovery by increasing blood flow to the targeted areas. This increased circulation helps to flush out metabolic waste products and deliver oxygen and nutrients to the muscles, promoting faster recovery and reducing muscle soreness.

3. **Reduced Muscle Tension and Pain**: Foam rolling can help alleviate muscle tension and pain caused by prolonged sitting or repetitive movements. By applying pressure to tight areas, you can release knots and trigger points, reducing discomfort and promoting relaxation.

4. **Improved Posture and Alignment**: Regular foam rolling can help correct postural imbalances and improve overall alignment. By targeting specific muscles that may be tight or overactive, you can restore balance and promote proper posture, reducing the risk of injuries and enhancing your overall physical appearance.

5. **Stress Relief**: Foam rolling can also provide stress relief and promote relaxation. The rhythmic movements and pressure applied during foam rolling can help calm the nervous system, reducing stress and promoting a sense of well-being.

Incorporating Foam Rolling into Your Fitness Routine

To incorporate foam rolling into your fitness routine, follow these steps:

1. **Choose the Right Foam Roller**: There are different types of foam rollers available, ranging from soft to firm. Beginners may prefer a softer foam roller, while those who are more experienced or have denser muscle tissue may benefit from a firmer roller. Experiment with different options to find the one that suits your needs.

2. **Warm Up**: Before starting your foam rolling session, it's important to warm up your muscles. Perform some light cardio exercises or dynamic stretches to increase blood flow and prepare your body for the foam rolling movements.

3. **Target Specific Areas**: Identify the areas of your body that feel tight or tense. Common areas to target include the calves, hamstrings, quadriceps, glutes, back, and shoulders. Roll slowly over each area, applying gentle pressure and pausing on any tender spots.

4. **Apply Pressure**: When foam rolling, it's important to apply enough pressure to feel a slight discomfort, but not to the point of pain. Use your body weight to control the intensity of the pressure. If an area is particularly sensitive, you can modify the pressure by using your hands or adjusting the position of your body.

5. **Roll Slowly**: Roll the foam roller slowly over the targeted area, focusing on the muscle belly rather than the joints or bony areas. Aim for a smooth and controlled movement, avoiding any sudden or jerky motions.

6. **Breathe and Relax**: As you foam roll, remember to breathe deeply and relax your body. Deep breathing can help release tension and promote relaxation, enhancing the effectiveness of the foam rolling session.

7. **Be Consistent**: To experience the full benefits of foam rolling, consistency is key. Aim to incorporate foam rolling into your fitness routine at least two to three times per week. As you become more familiar with the technique, you can increase the frequency or duration of your foam rolling sessions.

Key Foam Rolling Techniques

Here are some key foam rolling techniques to target specific areas of the body:

1. **Calves**: Sit on the floor with your legs extended and place the foam roller under your calves. Lift your hips off the ground and roll from the ankles to just below the knees.

2. **Hamstrings**: Sit on the foam roller with your legs extended and place your hands behind you for support. Roll from the glutes to just above the back of the knees, focusing on any tight or tender spots.

3. **Quadriceps**: Lie face down with the foam roller positioned under your thighs. Use your forearms to support your upper body and roll from the hips to just above the knees.

4. **Glutes**: Sit on the foam roller with one ankle crossed over the opposite knee. Lean slightly to the side of the crossed leg and roll over the glute muscles, focusing on any areas of tension.

5. **Back**: Lie on your back with the foam roller positioned under your mid-back. Support your head with your hands and gently roll from the mid-back to the upper back, focusing on any tight or tender spots.

Remember to adjust the techniques based on your comfort level and individual needs. If you have any pre-existing injuries or medical conditions, consult with a healthcare professional before incorporating foam rolling into your routine.

Foam rolling and self-myofascial release can be powerful tools for working women to enhance their fitness journey. By incorporating these techniques into your routine, you can improve flexibility, reduce muscle tension, and promote overall well-being. So grab a foam roller, set aside some time, and start reaping the benefits of foam rolling today!

Workout Recovery and Injury Prevention

8.1 Understanding the Importance of Recovery

In our fast-paced and demanding world, it's easy to get caught up in the hustle and bustle of work and fitness. As a working woman, you may find yourself constantly juggling multiple responsibilities and pushing yourself to achieve more. While this drive and determination are admirable, it's essential to understand the importance of recovery in maintaining a healthy work-life balance and achieving optimal performance in both your professional and fitness endeavors.

Recovery is a crucial component of any successful fitness routine. It refers to the period of time when your body repairs and adapts to the stress placed on it during exercise. Without adequate recovery, you risk overtraining, burnout, and even injury. As a working woman, it's vital to prioritize recovery to ensure you can continue to perform at your best and avoid the negative consequences of overexertion.

One of the primary reasons recovery is so important is that it allows your body to repair and rebuild itself. When you engage in physical activity, whether it's intense strength training or cardiovascular exercise, you create micro-tears in your muscles. These micro-tears are a normal part of the muscle-building process, but they need time to heal. During the recovery period, your body repairs these tears, making your muscles stronger and more resilient.

Additionally, recovery plays a crucial role in preventing injuries. When you push your body too hard without giving it adequate time to recover, you increase the risk of overuse injuries, such as tendonitis or stress fractures. These injuries can be debilitating and may require significant time off from both work and fitness activities. By incorporating proper recovery strategies into your routine, you can minimize the risk of injury and ensure long-term success in your fitness journey.

Another essential aspect of recovery is rest and sleep. As a working woman, you likely have a busy schedule, and it can be tempting to sacrifice sleep to fit everything in. However, sleep is a critical component of recovery and overall well-being. During sleep, your body releases growth hormone, which aids in muscle repair and recovery. It also allows your brain to process and consolidate information, improving cognitive function and decision-making abilities.

Lack of sleep can have detrimental effects on both your physical and mental health. It can lead to decreased immune function, increased stress levels, and impaired cognitive performance. To prioritize recovery, aim for seven to nine hours of quality sleep each night. Establish a consistent sleep schedule, create a relaxing bedtime routine, and create a sleep-friendly environment by keeping your bedroom cool, dark, and quiet.

Nutrition also plays a significant role in recovery. After a workout, your body needs the right nutrients to replenish glycogen stores, repair muscle tissue, and support overall recovery. Consuming a balanced meal or snack that includes carbohydrates, protein, and healthy fats within the first hour after exercise can help optimize recovery. Additionally, staying hydrated is crucial for proper recovery, as water is essential for transporting nutrients to your muscles and removing waste products.

Incorporating active recovery into your routine can also be beneficial. Active recovery refers to engaging in low-intensity activities that promote blood flow and help flush out metabolic waste products from your muscles. Examples of active recovery include light jogging, swimming, or gentle yoga. These activities can help reduce muscle soreness, improve flexibility, and enhance overall recovery.

Lastly, it's important to listen to your body and give yourself permission to rest when needed. As a working woman, it's easy to fall into the trap of feeling guilty for taking time off or prioritizing rest. However, rest is not a sign of weakness but rather a necessary part of the process. If you're feeling excessively fatigued, experiencing persistent muscle soreness, or noticing a decline in performance, it may be a sign that you need to take a rest day or incorporate more recovery into your routine.

In conclusion, understanding the importance of recovery is crucial for any working woman striving to balance work and fitness. Prioritizing recovery allows your body to repair and rebuild, prevents injuries, and promotes overall well-being. By incorporating strategies such as rest and sleep, proper nutrition, active recovery, and listening to your body, you can optimize your recovery and achieve long-term success in both your professional and fitness endeavors. Remember, recovery is not a luxury but a necessity for maintaining a healthy and sustainable lifestyle.

8.2 Rest and Sleep for Optimal Performance

Rest and sleep are often overlooked aspects of a fitness routine, especially for busy working women. However, they are crucial for optimal performance and overall well-being. In this section, we will explore the importance of rest and sleep, how they impact your fitness goals, and strategies to improve the quality of your rest and sleep.

The Importance of Rest

Rest is an essential component of any fitness program. It allows your body to recover and repair itself after intense workouts. When you exercise, you create micro-tears in your muscles, and rest is what allows them to heal and grow stronger. Without adequate rest, you risk overtraining, which can lead to fatigue, decreased performance, and even injuries.

Rest also plays a vital role in regulating your hormones and maintaining a healthy metabolism. When you don't get enough rest, your body produces more cortisol, a stress hormone that can hinder your weight loss efforts and increase your risk of developing chronic conditions like diabetes and heart disease.

The Power of Sleep

Sleep is equally important for your overall health and fitness. During sleep, your body goes through various stages of restorative processes that are essential for physical and mental well-being. These processes include tissue repair, muscle growth, hormone regulation, and memory consolidation.

Lack of sleep can have a significant impact on your fitness goals. It can lead to decreased energy levels, impaired cognitive function, increased appetite, and reduced motivation to exercise. Additionally, inadequate sleep can disrupt your body's ability to regulate insulin, leading to weight gain and an increased risk of developing metabolic disorders.

Strategies for Improving Rest and Sleep

Now that we understand the importance of rest and sleep let's explore some strategies to help you improve the quality of your rest and sleep:

1. Establish a Consistent Sleep Schedule Try to go to bed and wake up at the same time every day, even on weekends. This helps regulate your body's internal clock and promotes better sleep quality. Aim for 7-9 hours of sleep each night to ensure you are getting enough rest.

2. Create a Relaxing Bedtime Routine Develop a relaxing routine before bed to signal to your body that it's time to wind down. This could include activities such as reading a book, taking a warm bath, practicing meditation or deep breathing exercises, or listening to calming music. Avoid stimulating activities like using electronic devices or watching TV right before bed, as the blue light emitted from screens can interfere with your sleep.

3. Create a Sleep-Friendly Environment Make your bedroom a sleep-friendly environment by keeping it cool, dark, and quiet. Invest in comfortable bedding and a supportive mattress to ensure optimal comfort. Consider using blackout curtains, earplugs, or a white noise machine to block out any external disturbances that may disrupt your sleep.

4. Limit Caffeine and Alcohol Intake Caffeine and alcohol can interfere with your sleep quality. Limit your caffeine intake, especially in the afternoon and evening, as it can stay in your system for several hours. Similarly, while alcohol may initially make you feel drowsy, it can disrupt your sleep patterns and lead to poor sleep quality.

5. Manage Stress and Anxiety Stress and anxiety can significantly impact your ability to rest and sleep. Practice stress management techniques such as mindfulness, meditation, or journaling to help calm your mind before bed. If you find that stress or anxiety is consistently affecting your sleep, consider seeking professional help or talking to a therapist.

6. Create a Comfortable Sleep Environment Invest in a comfortable mattress and pillows that support your body and align your spine properly. Choose bedding that feels soft and cozy to enhance your sleep experience. Experiment with different sleep positions to find the one that works best for you in terms of comfort and reducing any potential pain or discomfort.

7. Avoid Heavy Meals and Stimulating Activities Before Bed Eating heavy meals close to bedtime can disrupt your sleep and cause discomfort. Try to finish your last meal at least two to three hours before bed. Additionally, avoid engaging in stimulating activities like intense exercise or work-related tasks right before bed, as they can make it harder for you to relax and fall asleep.

8. Consider Natural Sleep Aids If you are struggling with sleep, you may consider natural sleep aids such as herbal teas (chamomile, lavender), melatonin supplements, or aromatherapy with essential oils like lavender or valerian. However, it's important to consult with a healthcare professional before trying any sleep aids to ensure they are safe and suitable for you.

Conclusion

Rest and sleep are essential components of a balanced fitness routine for working women. Prioritizing rest and sleep will not only improve your physical performance but also enhance your overall well-being. By implementing the strategies discussed in this section, you can optimize your rest and sleep, allowing you to achieve your fitness goals while maintaining a healthy work-life balance. Remember, quality rest and sleep are the secret ingredients to unlock your full potential and power hustle.

8.3 Nutrition for Recovery

Proper nutrition plays a crucial role in the recovery process after intense workouts. As a busy working woman, it's important to fuel your body with the right nutrients to optimize your recovery and ensure that you can continue to perform at your best. In this section, we will explore the key principles of nutrition for recovery and provide practical tips to help you incorporate them into your daily routine.

The Importance of Post-Workout Nutrition

After a workout, your body needs to replenish its energy stores and repair damaged muscle tissues. This is where post-workout nutrition comes into play. Consuming the right nutrients within the optimal time frame can enhance your recovery, reduce muscle soreness, and promote muscle growth.

Macronutrients for Recovery Protein, carbohydrates, and fats are the three macronutrients that your body needs for optimal recovery. Let's take a closer look at each of them:

1. **Protein**: Protein is essential for repairing and rebuilding muscle tissues. Aim to consume a serving of high-quality protein within 30 minutes to an hour after your workout. Good sources of protein include lean meats, poultry, fish, eggs, dairy products, legumes, and plant-based protein powders.

2. **Carbohydrates**: Carbohydrates are your body's primary source of energy. Consuming carbohydrates after a workout helps replenish glycogen stores and provides the energy needed for muscle repair. Opt for complex carbohydrates such as whole grains, fruits, vegetables, and legumes.

3. **Fats**: While fats are not as critical immediately after a workout, they play a crucial role in overall health and should be included in your post-workout meals. Focus on consuming healthy fats such as avocados, nuts, seeds, and olive oil.

Hydration for Recovery Proper hydration is often overlooked but is essential for optimal recovery. During exercise, you lose fluids through sweat, and it's important to replenish them to maintain proper bodily functions. Aim to drink water before, during, and after your workout to stay hydrated. If you engage in intense or prolonged exercise, consider consuming a sports drink that contains electrolytes to replenish lost minerals.

Practical Tips for Nutrition and Recovery

Now that we understand the importance of post-workout nutrition let's explore some practical tips to help you incorporate it into your busy schedule:

1. **Plan Ahead**: Prepare your post-workout meals and snacks in advance to ensure that you have nutritious options readily available. Consider batch cooking and storing meals in portion-sized containers for easy grab-and-go options.

2. **Protein Smoothies**: Protein smoothies are a convenient and delicious way to replenish your body with essential nutrients. Blend together a combination of protein powder, fruits, vegetables, and a liquid of your choice for a quick and nutritious post-workout snack.

3. **Snack Smart**: Choose nutrient-dense snacks that provide a balance of protein, carbohydrates, and healthy fats. Some examples include Greek yogurt with berries, a handful of nuts and dried fruits, or a protein bar.

4. **Include Anti-Inflammatory Foods**: Incorporate foods with anti-inflammatory properties into your post-workout meals to reduce muscle inflammation and promote recovery. Examples include fatty fish (salmon, mackerel), turmeric, ginger, leafy greens, and berries.

5. **Listen to Your Body**: Pay attention to your body's hunger and fullness cues. Eat when you're hungry and stop when you're satisfied. This will help ensure that you're providing your body with the right amount of nutrients for recovery.

6. **Supplement Wisely**: While it's best to get your nutrients from whole foods, supplements can be a convenient option for busy individuals. Consult with a healthcare professional or registered dietitian to determine if any specific supplements may benefit your recovery.

7. **Avoid Excessive Alcohol and Caffeine**: Both alcohol and excessive caffeine consumption can interfere with your body's recovery process. Limit your intake of these substances, especially immediately after a workout.

Remember, nutrition for recovery is not just about what you eat immediately after a workout. It's about maintaining a balanced and nutritious diet throughout the day. Ensure that you're consuming a variety of whole foods that provide the necessary nutrients for optimal recovery and overall health.

By prioritizing post-workout nutrition and making conscious choices about the foods you consume, you can enhance your recovery, reduce muscle soreness, and continue to perform at your best as a busy working woman.

8.4 Preventing and Managing Injuries

Injuries can be a major setback when it comes to maintaining a consistent exercise routine. As a working woman, it's important to prioritize injury prevention and learn how to effectively manage any injuries that may occur. By taking proactive steps to prevent injuries and knowing how to handle them if they do happen, you can ensure that your fitness journey remains on track. In this section, we will explore some key strategies for preventing and managing injuries.

Understanding Common Exercise Injuries

Before we dive into prevention and management strategies, it's important to have a basic understanding of the most common exercise-related injuries. Some of the most prevalent injuries among women include sprains, strains, tendinitis, stress fractures, and muscle imbalances. These injuries can occur due to various factors such as overuse, improper form, inadequate warm-up, or pushing yourself too hard without allowing for proper recovery.

Warm-up and Cool-down

One of the most effective ways to prevent injuries is by incorporating a proper warm-up and cool-down routine into your exercise regimen. A warm-up helps to increase blood flow to your muscles, improve flexibility, and prepare your body for the upcoming workout. It should include dynamic stretches and movements that mimic the exercises you will be performing.

Similarly, a cool-down is essential for gradually bringing your heart rate and body temperature back to normal. It should include static stretches that target the muscles you worked during your workout. By taking the time to warm up and cool down properly, you can significantly reduce the risk of muscle strains and other injuries.

Listen to Your Body

As a working woman, it's easy to get caught up in the hustle and bustle of daily life. However, it's crucial to listen to your body and pay attention to any warning signs of potential injuries. If you experience persistent pain, discomfort, or unusual sensations during or after exercise, it's important to address them promptly.

Ignoring these warning signs can lead to more serious injuries and longer recovery times. If you're unsure about the severity of your symptoms, it's always a good idea to consult with a healthcare professional or a qualified fitness trainer who can provide guidance and support.

Proper Form and Technique

Maintaining proper form and technique during exercise is essential for preventing injuries. Whether you're lifting weights, performing bodyweight exercises, or engaging in cardiovascular activities, it's important to focus on your form and ensure that you're using the correct technique.

Improper form can put unnecessary stress on your joints, muscles, and ligaments, increasing the risk of injury. If you're unsure about the proper form for a particular exercise, consider working with a certified personal trainer who can guide you and help you perform the exercises correctly.

Gradual Progression

When it comes to exercise, it's important to progress gradually and avoid pushing yourself too hard, too soon. Rapidly increasing the intensity, duration, or frequency of your workouts can put excessive strain on your body, leading to overuse injuries.

Instead, focus on gradually increasing the intensity or duration of your workouts over time. This allows your body to adapt and build strength without placing excessive stress on your muscles and joints. Remember, consistency and patience are key when it comes to achieving long-term fitness goals.

Cross-Training and Rest Days

Incorporating cross-training and rest days into your exercise routine is crucial for injury prevention and overall recovery. Cross-training involves engaging in a variety of different activities to work different muscle groups and reduce the risk of overuse injuries.

Additionally, rest days are essential for giving your body time to recover and repair itself. Pushing through fatigue and ignoring the need for rest can lead to burnout and increased susceptibility to injuries. Aim to have at least one or two rest days per week to allow your body to recharge and heal.

Managing Injuries

Despite our best efforts, injuries can still occur. If you do find yourself dealing with an injury, it's important to take the necessary steps to manage it effectively. Here are some general guidelines for managing common exercise-related injuries:

1. **Rest and Ice**: Rest the injured area and apply ice for 15-20 minutes every 2-3 hours to reduce inflammation and pain.

2. **Compression and Elevation**: Use compression bandages to support the injured area and elevate it above heart level to reduce swelling.

3. **Pain Management**: Over-the-counter pain relievers can help manage pain and inflammation. However, it's important to consult with a healthcare professional before taking any medication.

4. **Seek Professional Help**: If the injury is severe or persists for an extended period, it's important to seek medical attention from a healthcare professional or a sports medicine specialist.

5. **Rehabilitation and Physical Therapy**: Depending on the nature and severity of the injury, rehabilitation exercises and physical therapy may be necessary to regain strength, flexibility, and function.

Remember, everyone's body is unique, and injuries can vary in severity. It's important to consult with a healthcare professional for personalized advice and guidance when it comes to managing injuries.

By prioritizing injury prevention strategies, listening to your body, and taking appropriate action when injuries occur, you can ensure that your fitness journey remains safe and sustainable. Remember, your health and well-being should always be the top priority, and taking care of your body will ultimately support your success in both work and fitness.

Work-Life Integration

9.1 Creating Boundaries and Setting Priorities

As a working woman, finding the balance between work and fitness can be a challenge. It often feels like there are not enough hours in the day to accomplish everything on your to-do list. However, by creating boundaries and setting priorities, you can effectively manage your time and make room for both work and fitness in your life.

The Importance of Boundaries

Setting boundaries is crucial for maintaining a healthy work-life balance. Without clear boundaries, it becomes easy for work to spill over into your personal life, leaving little time for self-care and fitness. By establishing boundaries, you are creating a structure that allows you to prioritize your well-being and make time for the activities that are important to you.

Define Your Non-Negotiables

Start by identifying your non-negotiables – the activities or commitments that are essential to your well-being. This could include regular exercise, spending quality time with loved ones, or engaging in hobbies that bring you joy. Once you have identified these non-negotiables, make a conscious effort to protect that time and prioritize them in your schedule.

Set Clear Work Hours

One effective way to create boundaries is by setting clear work hours. Determine the hours during which you will be fully dedicated to work, and communicate this to your colleagues and clients. By establishing these boundaries, you are signaling that you are not available outside of those designated work hours unless

it is an emergency. This allows you to have dedicated time for yourself and your
fitness activities.

Learn to Say No

Learning to say no is a powerful skill that can help you create boundaries and
protect your time. It's important to recognize that you don't have to say yes to
every request or opportunity that comes your way. Prioritize your commitments
and only take on tasks that align with your goals and values. By saying no to
things that don't serve you, you are freeing up time and energy for the things
that truly matter.

Delegate and Outsource

Another way to create boundaries is by delegating or outsourcing tasks that can
be done by others. As a working woman, it's important to recognize that you
don't have to do everything yourself. Identify tasks that can be handed off to
colleagues, family members, or hired professionals. By offloading some of your
responsibilities, you can free up time for fitness and self-care.

Time Blocking

Time blocking is a powerful technique that can help you prioritize your tasks and
make the most of your time. Start by identifying the most important activities
that need to be accomplished each day, both for work and fitness. Then, allocate
specific blocks of time in your schedule for each task. This helps you stay focused
and ensures that you have dedicated time for both work and fitness.

Avoid Multitasking

While multitasking may seem like an efficient way to get more done, it often
leads to decreased productivity and increased stress. Instead of trying to do
multiple things at once, focus on one task at a time. This allows you to give
your full attention to each activity and complete it more efficiently. By avoiding
multitasking, you can create boundaries between work and fitness and fully
immerse yourself in each activity.

Practice Self-Discipline

Creating boundaries and setting priorities requires self-discipline. It's important
to stay committed to your non-negotiables and resist the temptation to constantly
check work emails or take on additional tasks. Practice self-discipline by setting
clear boundaries and sticking to them. Remind yourself of the importance of
work-life balance and the benefits that come from prioritizing your well-being.

Communicate Your Boundaries

Lastly, it's important to communicate your boundaries to those around you. Let your colleagues, friends, and family members know about your work hours and the importance of your fitness activities. By communicating your boundaries, you are setting clear expectations and encouraging others to respect your time and priorities.

Remember, creating boundaries and setting priorities is a continuous process. It requires regular evaluation and adjustment as your circumstances change. By consistently prioritizing your well-being and making time for fitness, you can achieve a harmonious balance between work and personal life.

9.2 Building a Supportive Network

As a working woman striving to balance work and fitness, having a supportive network can make a world of difference in your journey. Building a network of like-minded individuals who understand and support your goals can provide you with the encouragement, motivation, and accountability you need to stay on track. In this section, we will explore the importance of building a supportive network and provide you with practical tips on how to do so.

The Power of a Supportive Network

A supportive network can be a game-changer when it comes to achieving your work and fitness goals. Here are a few reasons why building a supportive network is crucial:

1. **Encouragement and Motivation**: Surrounding yourself with individuals who share similar goals and aspirations can provide you with the encouragement and motivation you need to keep going, especially during challenging times. They can remind you of your capabilities and push you to reach new heights.

2. **Accountability**: A supportive network can help hold you accountable for your actions and commitments. When you have others who are invested in your success, you are more likely to stay committed and follow through on your fitness routines and work-related tasks.

3. **Knowledge and Resources**: Your network can be a valuable source of knowledge and resources. By connecting with individuals who have expertise in different areas, you can gain insights, tips, and advice that can enhance your work and fitness journey.

4. **Opportunities for Collaboration**: Building a supportive network opens doors to potential collaborations and partnerships. By connecting with like-minded individuals, you can explore opportunities to work together, share ideas, and learn from one another.

Tips for Building a Supportive Network

Now that you understand the importance of a supportive network, let's explore some practical tips to help you build one:

1. **Identify Your Needs**: Start by identifying what you need from a supportive network. Are you looking for workout buddies, mentors, or individuals who share similar career aspirations? Understanding your needs will help you focus your efforts on finding the right people.

2. **Join Fitness Communities**: Look for fitness communities or groups in your area that align with your interests and goals. This could be a local gym, a running club, or an online fitness community. Engage with the members, attend group workouts or events, and build connections with individuals who share your passion for fitness.

3. **Attend Networking Events**: Seek out networking events related to your industry or interests. These events provide an excellent opportunity to meet like-minded professionals who can support you in your career goals. Be open to initiating conversations, exchanging contact information, and following up with individuals you connect with.

4. **Utilize Social Media**: Social media platforms can be powerful tools for building a supportive network. Join fitness-related groups, follow fitness influencers, and engage with their content. Participate in discussions, ask questions, and connect with individuals who inspire you. Remember to be genuine and supportive in your interactions.

5. **Seek Mentors**: Mentors can provide guidance, support, and valuable insights based on their own experiences. Look for individuals who have achieved success in your field or have a strong fitness background. Reach out to them, express your admiration, and ask if they would be open to mentoring you. Remember to be respectful of their time and show gratitude for their support.

6. **Be a Supportive Network Member**: Building a supportive network is a two-way street. Show genuine interest in others' goals and aspirations, offer support and encouragement, and be willing to share your own knowledge and experiences. By being a valuable member of your network, you will attract like-minded individuals who are eager to support you in return.

7. **Attend Workshops and Seminars**: Look for workshops and seminars that align with your interests and professional development. These events not only provide opportunities to learn and grow but also allow you to connect with individuals who share similar goals and passions.

8. **Nurture Relationships**: Building a supportive network is not just about making connections; it's about nurturing and maintaining those relationships. Stay in touch with your network members, offer support

when needed, and celebrate each other's successes. Regularly check in with your network and make an effort to meet up or connect virtually.

Remember, building a supportive network takes time and effort. Be patient and persistent in your efforts, and don't be afraid to step out of your comfort zone. Surrounding yourself with individuals who believe in you and your goals will empower you to achieve a successful work and fitness balance.

Conclusion

Building a supportive network is a crucial aspect of balancing work and fitness as a working woman. Your network can provide you with the encouragement, motivation, accountability, knowledge, and opportunities for collaboration that are essential for your success. By following the tips provided in this section, you can start building a network of like-minded individuals who will support and empower you on your journey. Remember, your network is not just about what you can gain but also about what you can contribute. Be an active and supportive member, and watch your network flourish.

9.3 Finding Work-Life Balance

Finding a balance between work and life is a common struggle for many women. The demands of a career, family, and personal well-being can often feel overwhelming and leave little time for self-care and exercise. However, it is essential to prioritize finding work-life balance to maintain overall health and well-being. In this section, we will explore strategies and tips to help you find that balance and create a fulfilling and sustainable lifestyle.

Prioritizing Self-Care

One of the key components of achieving work-life balance is prioritizing self-care. Self-care involves taking intentional actions to nurture your physical, mental, and emotional well-being. It is crucial to recognize that self-care is not selfish but rather a necessary practice to maintain your overall health and happiness.

To prioritize self-care, start by identifying activities that bring you joy and relaxation. This could include activities such as reading, taking a bath, practicing yoga, or spending time with loved ones. Make a conscious effort to schedule regular self-care activities into your routine, just as you would schedule a work meeting or appointment. By prioritizing self-care, you are investing in your own well-being, which will ultimately benefit all areas of your life, including your work and fitness goals.

Setting Boundaries

Setting boundaries is another essential aspect of finding work-life balance. Boundaries help establish limits and create a sense of control over your time and energy.

Without clear boundaries, it is easy to become overwhelmed and feel like you are constantly juggling multiple responsibilities.

Start by defining your non-negotiables and identifying what is most important to you. This could include setting specific work hours, designating time for exercise, or establishing technology-free zones. Communicate your boundaries to your colleagues, friends, and family, and be firm in enforcing them. Remember that it is okay to say no and prioritize your well-being.

Time Management Strategies

Effective time management is crucial for finding work-life balance. By managing your time efficiently, you can allocate dedicated time for work, fitness, and personal activities. Here are some strategies to help you manage your time effectively:

1. Prioritize tasks: Start each day by identifying the most important tasks that need to be accomplished. Focus on completing these tasks first before moving on to less critical ones.

2. Delegate and outsource: Learn to delegate tasks that can be done by others. Whether it's at work or home, delegating tasks can free up valuable time for you to focus on what truly matters.

3. Time blocking: Allocate specific time blocks for different activities. For example, set aside dedicated time for work, exercise, family, and personal activities. Stick to these time blocks as much as possible to create a structured routine.

4. Avoid multitasking: Contrary to popular belief, multitasking can actually decrease productivity. Instead, focus on one task at a time and give it your full attention. This will help you complete tasks more efficiently and reduce stress.

5. Learn to say no: It's important to recognize your limits and not overcommit yourself. Practice saying no to tasks or activities that do not align with your priorities or values.

Creating a Supportive Network

Building a supportive network is crucial for maintaining work-life balance. Surrounding yourself with like-minded individuals who understand and support your goals can provide the encouragement and motivation needed to stay on track. Here are some ways to create a supportive network:

1. Find a workout buddy: Having a workout buddy can make exercise more enjoyable and help keep you accountable. Find a friend, colleague, or family member who shares your fitness goals and schedule regular workout sessions together.

2. Join fitness communities: Look for local fitness groups, classes, or online communities where you can connect with others who have similar interests. These communities can provide a sense of belonging and support as you navigate your fitness journey.

3. Seek mentorship: Find a mentor who has successfully achieved work-life balance and can provide guidance and advice. Having someone to turn to for support and guidance can be invaluable in maintaining balance and overcoming challenges.

4. Communicate with your loved ones: Openly communicate with your loved ones about your goals and the importance of work-life balance. Seek their understanding and support, and involve them in your journey whenever possible.

Embracing Flexibility

Work-life balance is not a one-size-fits-all concept. It is essential to embrace flexibility and adapt your approach as needed. Recognize that there will be times when work demands more of your attention, and other times when personal or family commitments take precedence. Embracing flexibility allows you to navigate these different seasons of life without feeling overwhelmed or guilty.

Remember that work-life balance is a continuous journey, and it may require adjustments along the way. Be kind to yourself and celebrate small victories. By finding a balance that works for you, you can create a fulfilling and sustainable lifestyle that prioritizes both your work and fitness goals.

Finding work-life balance is crucial for maintaining overall well-being. By prioritizing self-care, setting boundaries, managing your time effectively, creating a supportive network, and embracing flexibility, you can achieve a fulfilling and sustainable lifestyle that allows you to thrive both personally and professionally. Remember, finding work-life balance is a continuous process, and it may require adjustments along the way. Stay committed to your goals and be open to adapting your approach as needed.

9.4 Maintaining Healthy Relationships

Maintaining healthy relationships is an essential aspect of work-life integration. As a working woman, it can be challenging to balance your professional responsibilities with your personal life, including your relationships with family, friends, and romantic partners. However, with some conscious effort and effective communication, you can nurture and sustain these relationships while pursuing your career and fitness goals.

Prioritize Communication

Communication is the foundation of any healthy relationship. It is crucial to prioritize open and honest communication with your loved ones. Let them know about your work commitments, fitness routine, and any challenges you may be facing. By keeping the lines of communication open, you can avoid misunderstandings and ensure that everyone is on the same page.

Set Boundaries

Setting boundaries is essential to maintain a healthy work-life balance and protect your relationships. Clearly define your limits and communicate them to your loved ones. Let them know when you need uninterrupted time for work or exercise, and establish designated times for quality time together. By setting boundaries, you can avoid feelings of resentment and ensure that both your work and personal life receive the attention they deserve.

Quality Over Quantity

As a busy working woman, it's important to remember that quality time spent with loved ones is more valuable than the quantity of time. Instead of focusing on the number of hours you spend together, prioritize making the most of the time you do have. Plan activities that allow you to connect on a deeper level, such as going for a walk, cooking together, or having meaningful conversations. By making these moments count, you can strengthen your relationships despite your busy schedule.

Be Present

When you are with your loved ones, make a conscious effort to be fully present. Put away distractions such as your phone or work-related thoughts and give your undivided attention to the people you are with. Active listening and engaging in meaningful conversations will not only deepen your relationships but also show your loved ones that they are a priority in your life.

Support Each Other's Goals

Just as you have career and fitness goals, your loved ones may have their own aspirations as well. Show your support by actively encouraging and celebrating their achievements. Take an interest in their passions and offer assistance whenever possible. By being each other's cheerleaders, you can create a supportive environment that fosters personal growth and strengthens your relationships.

Plan Quality Time

In the midst of a busy schedule, it's important to intentionally plan quality time with your loved ones. Schedule regular date nights, family outings, or friend get-togethers to ensure that you have dedicated time to connect and bond. By making these plans in advance, you can prioritize your relationships and avoid the risk of neglecting them due to work or other commitments.

Practice Empathy and Understanding

Empathy and understanding are crucial in maintaining healthy relationships. Recognize that everyone has their own challenges and responsibilities, and be empathetic towards the demands they face. Understand that there may be times when work or fitness commitments take precedence, and be understanding of each other's needs. By practicing empathy, you can create a supportive and compassionate environment that strengthens your relationships.

Seek Support

As a working woman, it's important to recognize that you can't do it all alone. Seek support from your loved ones when you need it. Whether it's asking for help with household chores, childcare, or simply venting about a stressful day, reaching out to your support system can alleviate some of the burdens and strengthen your relationships. Remember, asking for help is not a sign of weakness but a testament to your strength in recognizing your limitations.

Prioritize Self-Care

Maintaining healthy relationships also requires taking care of yourself. Prioritize self-care to ensure that you have the energy and emotional capacity to invest in your relationships. Make time for activities that bring you joy and help you relax, such as reading, practicing mindfulness, or engaging in hobbies. By prioritizing self-care, you can show up as your best self in your relationships and avoid burnout.

Flexibility and Adaptability

Flexibility and adaptability are key when it comes to maintaining healthy relationships as a working woman. Recognize that there may be times when unexpected work demands arise or your fitness routine needs to be adjusted. Be willing to adapt and find alternative ways to spend quality time with your loved ones. By being flexible, you can navigate the challenges that arise and ensure that your relationships remain strong.

Remember, maintaining healthy relationships is a continuous effort that requires open communication, understanding, and prioritization. By investing time and energy into nurturing your relationships, you can create a harmonious work-life integration that supports both your career and personal life.

Staying Motivated and Consistent

10.1 Finding Your Inner Motivation

Motivation is the driving force behind any successful endeavor, and maintaining a consistent exercise routine is no exception. As a busy working woman, it can be challenging to find the motivation to prioritize your fitness goals amidst the demands of your career and personal life. However, by tapping into your inner motivation, you can overcome obstacles and stay committed to your health and well-being.

Understanding Motivation

Motivation is a complex psychological concept that can vary from person to person. It is the internal or external drive that compels us to take action towards achieving our goals. In the context of exercise, motivation plays a crucial role in sustaining a regular fitness routine. Understanding the different types of motivation can help you identify what drives you and how to harness it effectively.

Intrinsic Motivation Intrinsic motivation refers to the internal desire and enjoyment derived from engaging in an activity. When it comes to exercise, intrinsic motivation is fueled by the satisfaction, pleasure, and sense of accomplishment you experience during and after a workout. It is driven by your personal values, interests, and the positive feelings associated with being physically active.

To tap into your intrinsic motivation, reflect on the aspects of exercise that bring you joy and fulfillment. It could be the feeling of strength and empowerment, the sense of accomplishment after completing a challenging workout, or the mental clarity and stress relief that physical activity provides. By focusing on these intrinsic rewards, you can cultivate a deeper connection to your fitness journey.

Extrinsic Motivation Extrinsic motivation, on the other hand, is driven by external factors such as rewards, recognition, or social approval. It involves engaging in an activity to attain a specific outcome or avoid negative consequences. While extrinsic motivation can be helpful in initiating behavior change, it may not be as sustainable in the long run.

Common examples of extrinsic motivation for exercise include wanting to lose weight, fit into a certain dress size, or receive praise from others. While these external factors can provide initial motivation, they may not be enough to keep you consistently engaged in your fitness routine. It is important to recognize that true and lasting motivation comes from within.

Cultivating Inner Motivation

Finding your inner motivation requires self-reflection, goal-setting, and a deep understanding of your values and priorities. Here are some strategies to help you cultivate and maintain your inner motivation:

Set Meaningful Goals Setting meaningful and realistic goals is essential for staying motivated. Take the time to identify what you want to achieve through your fitness journey. Your goals should align with your values and be specific, measurable, attainable, relevant, and time-bound (SMART). For example, instead of setting a vague goal like "get fit," you could set a SMART goal like "run a 5K race in three months."

Find Your Why Understanding your "why" is crucial for sustaining motivation. Ask yourself why exercise is important to you and how it aligns with your values and aspirations. Your "why" could be related to your physical health, mental well-being, personal growth, or setting a positive example for your loved ones. When you have a clear understanding of your purpose, it becomes easier to stay committed, even when faced with challenges.

Create a Vision Board Visualizing your goals can be a powerful motivator. Consider creating a vision board that represents your fitness aspirations. Include images, quotes, and words that inspire and remind you of what you want to achieve. Place your vision board in a prominent location where you can see it daily, such as your bedroom or office. This visual reminder will help keep your goals at the forefront of your mind and reinforce your motivation.

Find an Accountability Partner Having someone to hold you accountable can significantly increase your motivation and commitment. Find a workout buddy or enlist the support of a friend, family member, or colleague who shares similar fitness goals. You can exercise together, check in regularly, and provide each other with encouragement and support. Knowing that someone is counting on you can be a powerful motivator to stay consistent.

Track Your Progress Tracking your progress is an effective way to stay motivated and celebrate your achievements. Keep a workout journal or use a fitness tracking app to record your workouts, track your progress, and monitor your improvements. Seeing how far you've come can boost your confidence and provide the motivation to keep pushing forward.

Mix Up Your Routine Monotony can dampen motivation, so it's important to keep your exercise routine fresh and exciting. Incorporate variety into your workouts by trying new activities, exploring different fitness classes, or challenging yourself with new goals. By keeping things interesting, you'll be more likely to stay engaged and motivated.

Practice Self-Compassion Remember to be kind to yourself throughout your fitness journey. It's normal to have setbacks or days when motivation is low. Instead of beating yourself up, practice self-compassion and focus on progress rather than perfection. Celebrate small victories and acknowledge the effort you put into taking care of your health and well-being.

Conclusion

Finding your inner motivation is key to maintaining a consistent exercise routine as a busy working woman. By understanding the different types of motivation and implementing strategies to cultivate your inner drive, you can overcome obstacles, stay committed to your fitness goals, and achieve a healthy work-life balance. Remember, motivation is not a finite resource but a skill that can be nurtured and strengthened over time.

10.2 Tracking Progress and Celebrating Milestones

Tracking your progress and celebrating milestones is an essential part of staying motivated and consistent in your fitness journey. It allows you to see how far you've come, stay accountable to your goals, and provides a sense of accomplishment. In this section, we will explore different methods of tracking progress and how to celebrate your milestones along the way.

The Importance of Tracking Progress

Tracking your progress is crucial because it provides tangible evidence of your hard work and dedication. It allows you to see the improvements you've made in various aspects of your fitness journey, such as strength, endurance, flexibility, and overall well-being. Here are some key benefits of tracking your progress:

1. **Motivation:** Seeing your progress can be incredibly motivating. It reminds you of the positive changes you've made and encourages you to keep pushing forward.

2. **Accountability:** Tracking your progress holds you accountable to your goals. It helps you stay focused and committed, as you can see whether you're on track or need to make adjustments.

3. **Identifying Patterns:** By tracking your progress, you can identify patterns and trends in your fitness journey. This allows you to make informed decisions about what works best for you and what areas need improvement.

4. **Setting Realistic Goals:** Tracking your progress helps you set realistic goals. By understanding where you currently stand, you can set achievable milestones that align with your capabilities and aspirations.

Methods of Tracking Progress

There are various methods you can use to track your progress. The key is to find a method that works best for you and aligns with your goals and preferences. Here are some popular methods:

1. **Fitness Journal:** Keeping a fitness journal allows you to record your workouts, track your progress, and note any challenges or successes along the way. You can include details such as the exercises you performed,

the number of sets and reps, and how you felt during the workout. This method provides a comprehensive overview of your fitness journey.

2. **Measurement and Body Composition:** Tracking your body measurements, such as waist circumference, hip circumference, and body fat percentage, can provide valuable insights into your progress. Take measurements regularly and compare them over time to see changes in your body composition.

3. **Progress Photos:** Progress photos are a visual representation of your journey. Take photos at regular intervals, such as every month or every few months, in the same lighting and clothing. Comparing these photos side by side can help you see the physical changes in your body.

4. **Fitness Apps and Wearable Devices:** There are numerous fitness apps and wearable devices available that can track your workouts, steps, heart rate, and other metrics. These tools provide real-time data and can sync with your smartphone or computer, making it easy to monitor your progress.

5. **Performance-Based Goals:** Setting performance-based goals, such as running a certain distance in a specific time or lifting a certain weight, allows you to track your progress based on your abilities and achievements. Keep a record of your personal bests and strive to improve them over time.

Celebrating Milestones

Celebrating milestones is an important part of your fitness journey. It not only acknowledges your hard work but also provides a sense of accomplishment and motivation to keep going. Here are some ways to celebrate your milestones:

1. **Reward Yourself:** Treat yourself to something special when you reach a milestone. It could be a massage, a new workout outfit, a spa day, or anything that brings you joy and makes you feel appreciated for your efforts.

2. **Share Your Success:** Share your achievements with friends, family, or your fitness community. Celebrating your milestones with others not only allows you to receive support and encouragement but also inspires and motivates those around you.

3. **Reflect and Appreciate:** Take time to reflect on your journey and appreciate how far you've come. Write in your journal or create a gratitude list, acknowledging the progress you've made and the positive changes you've experienced.

4. **Set New Goals:** Celebrating a milestone is an excellent opportunity to set new goals and challenge yourself further. Use your achievements as a stepping stone to reach even greater heights in your fitness journey.

5. **Plan a Fitness Event:** Organize a fitness event or participate in a race or competition to celebrate your milestone. It can be a fun way to challenge yourself and showcase your progress to others.

Remember, celebrating milestones is not just about the big achievements. It's also about acknowledging the small victories along the way. Every step forward, no matter how small, is worth celebrating.

Conclusion

Tracking your progress and celebrating milestones are essential components of a successful fitness journey. By tracking your progress, you can stay motivated, accountable, and make informed decisions about your goals. Celebrating milestones allows you to appreciate your hard work, reflect on your achievements, and set new challenges. Embrace the power of tracking and celebrating, and watch as your fitness journey becomes even more rewarding and fulfilling.

10.3 Accountability Strategies

Accountability is a crucial aspect of achieving any goal, especially when it comes to balancing work and fitness. As a busy working woman, it can be challenging to stay motivated and consistent with your exercise routine. That's where accountability strategies come into play. By implementing these strategies, you can hold yourself accountable and stay on track with your fitness goals. Let's explore some effective accountability strategies that can help you maintain your motivation and consistency.

Find an Accountability Partner

One of the most effective ways to stay accountable is by finding an accountability partner. This can be a friend, colleague, or family member who shares similar fitness goals or is also looking to maintain a healthy lifestyle. Having someone to check in with regularly can provide the necessary support and encouragement to keep you motivated. You can set specific goals together, share progress updates, and even work out together. Knowing that someone is counting on you can be a powerful motivator to stay consistent with your exercise routine.

Join a Fitness Community or Group

Another great way to stay accountable is by joining a fitness community or group. This can be a local gym, fitness class, or an online community of like-minded individuals. Being part of a community that shares similar goals and interests can provide a sense of belonging and support. You can participate in group challenges, share your progress, and seek advice from others who have faced similar challenges. The collective energy and motivation within a fitness community can help you stay on track and push through any obstacles.

Set Clear and Measurable Goals

Setting clear and measurable goals is essential for accountability. When your goals are specific and measurable, it becomes easier to track your progress and hold yourself accountable. Instead of setting vague goals like "exercise more," set specific goals like "exercise for 30 minutes, five days a week." Break down your goals into smaller milestones and celebrate each achievement along the way. By having clear goals, you can monitor your progress and make adjustments if needed to stay on track.

Create a Schedule and Stick to It

Creating a schedule and sticking to it is crucial for maintaining accountability. Treat your exercise routine as an important appointment that you cannot miss. Block out specific times in your calendar dedicated to exercise and treat them as non-negotiable. By prioritizing your workouts and treating them as essential as any other work commitment, you are more likely to stay consistent. Remember, consistency is key when it comes to achieving your fitness goals.

Use Technology and Apps

In today's digital age, there are numerous apps and technologies available to help you stay accountable. Fitness tracking apps, such as MyFitnessPal or Fitbit, can help you monitor your progress, track your workouts, and even connect with friends for added accountability. These apps can provide reminders, track your steps, calories burned, and even offer personalized workout plans. By leveraging technology, you can have a virtual accountability partner right at your fingertips.

Track Your Progress

Tracking your progress is an essential accountability strategy. Keep a record of your workouts, including the exercises performed, duration, and intensity. You can use a fitness journal, a spreadsheet, or even a mobile app to track your progress. Regularly reviewing your progress can help you identify patterns, areas of improvement, and celebrate your achievements. It also serves as a visual reminder of your commitment and can motivate you to keep pushing forward.

Reward Yourself

Rewarding yourself for reaching milestones and staying consistent can be a powerful motivator. Set up a reward system for yourself, where you treat yourself to something you enjoy after achieving a specific goal. It could be a spa day, a new workout outfit, or even a weekend getaway. By having something to look forward to, you are more likely to stay motivated and committed to your fitness routine.

Stay Positive and Practice Self-Compassion

Accountability is not about being hard on yourself or beating yourself up for any setbacks. It's about staying positive and practicing self-compassion. Understand that setbacks and plateaus are a natural part of any fitness journey. Instead of dwelling on them, focus on what you have accomplished and how far you have come. Be kind to yourself and acknowledge that progress takes time. By maintaining a positive mindset and practicing self-compassion, you can stay motivated and committed to your fitness goals.

Regularly Evaluate and Adjust

Lastly, regularly evaluate your accountability strategies and make adjustments as needed. What works for one person may not work for another. Be open to trying different strategies and see what resonates with you. If you find that a particular strategy is not effective, don't be afraid to switch it up and try something new. The key is to find what keeps you motivated and consistent in your fitness journey.

By implementing these accountability strategies, you can stay motivated and consistent in balancing work and fitness. Remember, accountability is a personal commitment to yourself and your well-being. Embrace the power of accountability and watch as it transforms your fitness journey.

10.4 Overcoming Plateaus and Setbacks

As you progress on your fitness journey, you may encounter plateaus and setbacks. These can be frustrating and demotivating, but it's important to remember that they are a normal part of any long-term endeavor. Plateaus occur when your progress stalls, and setbacks are temporary obstacles that hinder your progress. In this section, we will explore strategies to overcome plateaus and setbacks, so you can continue moving forward on your path to a balanced and healthy life.

Recognizing Plateaus

Plateaus can happen for various reasons. Your body may have adapted to your current exercise routine, or you may have reached a point where your progress naturally slows down. It's essential to recognize when you've hit a plateau so that you can take appropriate action to overcome it.

One way to identify a plateau is by tracking your progress. Keep a record of your workouts, including the exercises, sets, reps, and weights used. By reviewing this information, you can determine if you've been consistently performing the same routine without any improvements. Additionally, pay attention to how your body feels during workouts. If you no longer feel challenged or notice a lack of improvement in your strength or endurance, it may be a sign of a plateau.

Overcoming Plateaus

When faced with a plateau, it's crucial to reassess your approach and make necessary adjustments. Here are some strategies to help you overcome plateaus and continue making progress:

1. Change Your Workout Routine One of the most effective ways to break through a plateau is by changing your workout routine. Your body adapts to the stress placed upon it, so introducing new exercises, varying the intensity, or altering the order of your exercises can challenge your muscles in different ways. Consider incorporating different types of workouts, such as high-intensity interval training (HIIT), circuit training, or trying new fitness classes. By keeping your body guessing, you can stimulate new growth and progress.

2. Increase the Intensity If you've been performing the same exercises with the same weights and repetitions for an extended period, it may be time to increase the intensity. Gradually increase the weight you lift or the number of repetitions you perform. Pushing yourself outside your comfort zone can help you break through plateaus and continue making gains.

3. Focus on Progressive Overload Progressive overload is the principle of gradually increasing the demands placed on your body to continually make progress. This can be achieved by increasing the weight, the number of repetitions, or the intensity of your workouts over time. By consistently challenging your body, you can overcome plateaus and stimulate further growth.

4. Prioritize Recovery Sometimes, plateaus can be a result of overtraining or inadequate recovery. Ensure you are giving your body enough time to rest and recover between workouts. Incorporate rest days into your routine and prioritize sleep to allow your muscles to repair and grow. Additionally, pay attention to your nutrition and ensure you are fueling your body with the right nutrients to support recovery.

5. Seek Professional Guidance If you're struggling to overcome a plateau, consider seeking guidance from a fitness professional. They can assess your current routine, provide expert advice, and create a personalized plan to help you break through the plateau. A professional can also help you identify any potential form or technique issues that may be hindering your progress.

Dealing with Setbacks

Setbacks are temporary obstacles that can occur at any time during your fitness journey. They can be caused by various factors, such as injuries, illness, work-related stress, or personal challenges. While setbacks can be discouraging, it's important to approach them with a positive mindset and a plan for recovery. Here are some strategies to help you deal with setbacks:

1. Accept and Adapt The first step in overcoming setbacks is accepting that they happen and understanding that they are a normal part of life. Instead of dwelling on the setback, focus on adapting your routine to accommodate the situation. This may involve modifying your workouts, seeking alternative forms of exercise, or adjusting your goals temporarily.

2. Listen to Your Body During a setback, it's crucial to listen to your body and prioritize your health and well-being. If you're injured or unwell, pushing through may worsen the situation and prolong your recovery. Take the necessary time off to heal and consult with a healthcare professional if needed. Remember, setbacks are temporary, and your long-term health should always be the priority.

3. Set Realistic Expectations When recovering from a setback, it's important to set realistic expectations for yourself. Understand that progress may be slower during this time, and that's okay. Be patient with yourself and focus on small, achievable goals that align with your current capabilities. Celebrate each milestone, no matter how small, as it signifies progress and resilience.

4. Seek Support During setbacks, it can be helpful to seek support from friends, family, or a fitness community. Surrounding yourself with positive and understanding individuals can provide encouragement and motivation during challenging times. Share your experiences, seek advice, and lean on others for support when needed.

5. Stay Positive and Persistent Lastly, maintain a positive mindset and stay persistent. Setbacks are temporary roadblocks, and with time and effort, you can overcome them. Focus on the progress you've made so far and remind yourself of your long-term goals. Use setbacks as an opportunity to learn and grow, and remember that every setback is a stepping stone towards a stronger and more resilient you.

By implementing these strategies, you can overcome plateaus and setbacks, and continue progressing on your fitness journey. Remember, setbacks are not failures but opportunities for growth and resilience. Stay committed, stay motivated, and stay consistent, and you will achieve the balance between work and fitness that you desire.

Self-Care and Wellness Rituals

11.1 The Importance of Self-Care

In today's fast-paced and demanding world, it's easy for women to get caught up in the hustle and bustle of work and forget to take care of themselves. However, self-care is not a luxury; it is a necessity for maintaining overall well-being and achieving success in both work and fitness. In this section, we will explore the importance of self-care and how it can positively impact your life.

The Definition of Self-Care

Self-care is the practice of intentionally taking care of your physical, mental, and emotional well-being. It involves making choices that prioritize your health and happiness, allowing you to recharge and rejuvenate. Self-care is not selfish; it is an essential part of maintaining a healthy work-life balance and preventing burnout.

The Benefits of Self-Care

1. **Improved Physical Health**: Engaging in self-care activities such as regular exercise, eating nutritious meals, and getting enough sleep can significantly improve your physical health. Taking care of your body allows you to have more energy, better focus, and increased productivity in both your work and fitness endeavors.

2. **Enhanced Mental Well-being**: Self-care practices can have a profound impact on your mental health. Taking time for yourself, practicing mindfulness, and engaging in activities that bring you joy can reduce stress, anxiety, and depression. It promotes a positive mindset, boosts self-esteem, and improves overall mental well-being.

3. **Increased Productivity**: When you prioritize self-care, you are better equipped to handle the demands of work and fitness. By taking care of your physical and mental health, you can improve your focus, concentration, and problem-solving abilities. This, in turn, leads to increased productivity and efficiency in all areas of your life.

4. **Stress Reduction**: Self-care activities such as meditation, deep breathing exercises, and engaging in hobbies can help reduce stress levels. When you take time to relax and unwind, you give your body and mind a chance to recharge and recover from the daily stresses of work and life. This can lead to improved resilience and better stress management skills.

5. **Improved Relationships**: When you prioritize self-care, you are better able to show up as your best self in your relationships. Taking care of your own needs allows you to have more energy, patience, and compassion for others. It also sets a positive example for those around you, encouraging them to prioritize their own self-care.

Incorporating Self-Care into Your Routine

Now that you understand the importance of self-care, it's time to explore how you can incorporate it into your daily routine. Here are some practical tips to help you get started:

1. **Identify Your Needs**: Take some time to reflect on what activities bring you joy, relaxation, and rejuvenation. It could be anything from taking a bubble bath, reading a book, going for a walk in nature, or practicing yoga. Identify what self-care activities resonate with you and make a list of them.

2. **Schedule Self-Care Time**: Treat self-care as an essential appointment with yourself. Schedule dedicated time for self-care activities in your daily or weekly calendar. Treat this time as non-negotiable and prioritize it just like you would any other important commitment.

3. **Start Small**: Incorporating self-care into your routine doesn't have to be overwhelming. Start with small, manageable steps. It could be as simple as taking a few minutes each day to practice deep breathing or enjoying a cup of tea in the morning. Gradually increase the time and intensity of your self-care activities as you become more comfortable.

4. **Practice Mindfulness**: Mindfulness is the practice of being fully present in the moment. Incorporate mindfulness into your self-care routine by focusing on the sensations, thoughts, and emotions that arise during your chosen activity. This can help you cultivate a sense of gratitude and appreciation for the present moment.

5. **Set Boundaries**: Learn to say no to activities or commitments that drain your energy and take away from your self-care time. Setting boundaries is crucial for protecting your well-being and ensuring that you have enough time and energy to take care of yourself.

Remember, self-care is not a one-time event; it is an ongoing practice. It requires consistent effort and commitment to prioritize your well-being. By making self-care a priority, you will not only enhance your work and fitness journey but also improve your overall quality of life. So, take the time to nurture yourself, recharge your batteries, and embrace the power of self-care.

11.2 Creating a Personal Wellness Routine

Creating a personal wellness routine is essential for maintaining a healthy work-life balance and ensuring that you prioritize self-care. In today's fast-paced world, it can be easy to neglect our own well-being while juggling work responsibilities and other commitments. However, by intentionally carving out time for self-care and incorporating wellness practices into our daily lives, we can enhance our overall well-being and improve our ability to handle the demands of work and life.

The Importance of a Personal Wellness Routine

A personal wellness routine is a set of intentional practices that promote physical, mental, and emotional well-being. It is a way to prioritize self-care and ensure that you are taking care of yourself amidst the busyness of life. By creating a routine that includes activities such as exercise, mindfulness, healthy eating, and adequate rest, you can enhance your overall quality of life and improve your ability to handle stress.

Assessing Your Needs and Goals

Before creating your personal wellness routine, it's important to assess your needs and goals. Take some time to reflect on what areas of your life could benefit from more attention and care. Are you feeling physically exhausted? Do you struggle with stress and anxiety? Are you finding it challenging to maintain a healthy diet? Identifying your needs will help you tailor your routine to address those specific areas.

Next, set clear goals for your wellness routine. What do you hope to achieve through these practices? Your goals could be related to improving your fitness level, reducing stress, increasing energy levels, or enhancing your overall well-being. Having specific goals will give you direction and motivation as you create your routine.

Designing Your Personal Wellness Routine

When designing your personal wellness routine, it's important to consider your schedule and lifestyle. Find a balance between activities that you enjoy and those that are practical for your daily life. Here are some key components to include in your routine:

1. Exercise Regular exercise is crucial for maintaining physical health and managing stress. Choose activities that you enjoy and that align with your fitness goals. Whether it's going for a run, attending a yoga class, or lifting weights, aim for at least 150 minutes of moderate-intensity exercise per week. Schedule your workouts at times that work best for you, whether it's in the morning, during lunch breaks, or in the evening.

2. Mindfulness and Meditation Incorporating mindfulness and meditation into your routine can help reduce stress, improve focus, and enhance overall well-being. Set aside a few minutes each day for meditation or mindfulness practices such as deep breathing exercises or guided meditation apps. Find a quiet space where you can relax and be present in the moment.

3. Healthy Eating Nutrition plays a vital role in overall wellness. Plan and prepare nutritious meals and snacks that fuel your body and provide the energy you need to thrive. Include a variety of fruits, vegetables, whole grains, lean proteins, and healthy fats in your diet. Avoid processed foods and sugary drinks as much as possible. Consider meal prepping to save time and ensure that you have healthy options readily available.

4. Rest and Sleep Adequate rest and quality sleep are essential for physical and mental well-being. Aim for 7-9 hours of sleep each night and establish a consistent sleep schedule. Create a relaxing bedtime routine that helps you unwind and prepare for a restful night's sleep. Avoid electronic devices before bed and create a sleep-friendly environment in your bedroom.

5. Self-Care Activities Incorporate self-care activities into your routine to nurture your mental and emotional well-being. This could include activities such as reading, taking baths, practicing hobbies, journaling, or spending time in nature. Find activities that bring you joy and help you relax and recharge.

6. Social Connections Maintaining healthy relationships and social connections is an important aspect of overall wellness. Make time for meaningful interactions with friends, family, and loved ones. Schedule regular social activities or join clubs or groups that align with your interests. Surrounding yourself with positive and supportive people can greatly contribute to your well-being.

Implementing and Adjusting Your Routine

Once you have designed your personal wellness routine, it's time to implement it into your daily life. Start by incorporating one or two practices at a time and gradually build upon them. Consistency is key, so aim to stick to your routine as much as possible. However, be flexible and willing to adjust your routine as needed. Life can be unpredictable, and there may be times when you need to adapt your routine to accommodate unexpected events or changes in your schedule.

Conclusion

Creating a personal wellness routine is a powerful way to prioritize self-care and enhance your overall well-being. By assessing your needs, setting goals, and designing a routine that includes exercise, mindfulness, healthy eating, rest, self-care activities, and social connections, you can create a balanced and fulfilling life. Remember, your routine should be tailored to your unique needs and lifestyle. Embrace the power of self-care and make your personal wellness a priority.

11.3 Mindful Eating and Intuitive Living

In our fast-paced and busy lives, it's easy to fall into the trap of mindless eating and neglecting our body's needs. However, by practicing mindful eating and embracing intuitive living, we can develop a healthier relationship with food and nourish our bodies in a more balanced way. Mindful eating is about being present and fully engaged with the act of eating, while intuitive living involves listening to our body's cues and honoring its needs. Together, these practices can help us make better food choices, improve digestion, and enhance overall well-being.

The Power of Mindful Eating

Mindful eating is a practice that encourages us to slow down, pay attention, and savor each bite of food. By being fully present during meals, we can cultivate a deeper connection with our bodies and the food we consume. Here are some key principles of mindful eating:

1. **Eat with Awareness**: Instead of mindlessly consuming food while multi-tasking or watching TV, make an effort to eat without distractions. Focus on the flavors, textures, and smells of your food. Take the time to chew slowly and savor each bite.

2. **Listen to Your Body**: Tune in to your body's hunger and fullness cues. Eat when you're hungry and stop when you're satisfied, rather than eating until you're overly full. Pay attention to how different foods make you feel and adjust your choices accordingly.

3. **Engage Your Senses**: Engage all your senses while eating. Notice the colors, smells, and textures of your food. Take the time to appreciate the visual appeal of your meal and the aroma that wafts from it. This sensory experience can enhance your enjoyment and satisfaction.

4. **Practice Gratitude**: Cultivate a sense of gratitude for the food you have. Recognize the effort that went into growing, preparing, and serving your meal. This mindset of gratitude can help you develop a more positive relationship with food.

Intuitive Living: Honoring Your Body's Needs

Intuitive living is about listening to your body's signals and honoring its needs. It involves trusting your instincts and making choices that align with your physical and emotional well-being. Here are some ways to embrace intuitive living:

1. **Tune into Your Hunger and Fullness**: Pay attention to your body's hunger and fullness cues. Eat when you're hungry and stop when you're satisfied. Avoid restrictive diets or rigid eating schedules that disconnect you from your body's natural signals.

2. **Eat for Nourishment**: Choose foods that nourish your body and provide the energy and nutrients it needs. Focus on whole, unprocessed foods that are rich in vitamins, minerals, and fiber. Listen to your body's cravings and give yourself permission to enjoy a wide variety of foods in moderation.

3. **Embrace Pleasure and Satisfaction**: Food should be enjoyed, not just seen as fuel. Allow yourself to savor and enjoy the foods you love without guilt. When you eat mindfully and savor each bite, you can experience greater satisfaction and reduce the urge to overeat.

4. **Cultivate Self-Compassion**: Be kind to yourself and let go of judgment around food choices. Practice self-compassion and forgive yourself for any perceived "mistakes" or deviations from your ideal eating plan. Remember that balance and flexibility are key to long-term well-being.

Practical Tips for Mindful Eating and Intuitive Living

Here are some practical tips to help you incorporate mindful eating and intuitive living into your daily life:

1. **Create a Peaceful Eating Environment**: Set aside a designated space for meals that is free from distractions. Create a calm and inviting atmosphere that allows you to fully focus on your food and the act of eating.

2. **Slow Down and Chew Thoroughly**: Take your time to chew each bite thoroughly before swallowing. This not only aids digestion but also allows you to fully experience the flavors and textures of your food.

3. **Practice Portion Control**: Use smaller plates and bowls to help control portion sizes. Pay attention to your body's signals of fullness and avoid the temptation to overeat.

4. **Keep a Food Journal**: Consider keeping a food journal to track your eating habits and emotions associated with food. This can help you identify patterns and make more conscious choices.

5. **Engage in Mindful Movement**: Incorporate mindful movement practices such as yoga or walking into your routine. This can help you connect with your body and enhance your overall well-being.

Remember, mindful eating and intuitive living are not about perfection or strict rules. They are about developing a healthier and more balanced relationship with food and your body. By practicing these principles, you can nourish yourself both physically and emotionally, leading to a more fulfilling and empowered life.

11.4 Practicing Gratitude and Self-Reflection

In the hustle and bustle of our daily lives, it's easy to get caught up in the never-ending to-do lists and forget to take a moment for ourselves. However, practicing gratitude and self-reflection is an essential part of maintaining a healthy work-life balance and overall well-being. In this section, we will explore the power of gratitude and self-reflection and how they can positively impact your life as a working woman.

The Power of Gratitude

Gratitude is the practice of acknowledging and appreciating the good things in your life. It is a powerful tool that can shift your mindset from focusing on what you lack to recognizing and being thankful for what you have. As a working woman, cultivating a sense of gratitude can help you find joy and contentment amidst the challenges and demands of your professional and personal life.

Practicing gratitude has been scientifically proven to have numerous benefits for both mental and physical health. Research shows that regularly expressing gratitude can improve sleep quality, boost immune function, reduce stress levels, and increase overall happiness and life satisfaction. By incorporating gratitude into your daily routine, you can enhance your well-being and resilience, making it easier to navigate the ups and downs of work and life.

Ways to Practice Gratitude

There are many simple and effective ways to incorporate gratitude into your daily life. Here are a few practices you can try:

1. **Gratitude Journaling**: Set aside a few minutes each day to write down three things you are grateful for. It could be something as small as a delicious cup of coffee or as significant as a supportive colleague. By focusing on the positive aspects of your life, you can shift your mindset and cultivate a sense of appreciation.

2. **Gratitude Letters**: Take the time to write a heartfelt letter expressing your gratitude to someone who has made a positive impact on your life. It could be a mentor, a friend, or a family member. Not only will this practice deepen your connection with others, but it will also remind you of the support and love you have in your life.

3. **Gratitude Walks**: Incorporate gratitude into your exercise routine by going for a walk and consciously focusing on the things you are grateful for. Take in the beauty of nature, appreciate the small details around you, and reflect on the positive aspects of your life. This practice can help you feel more grounded and present.

4. **Gratitude Rituals**: Create a gratitude ritual that works for you. It could be lighting a candle and reflecting on your day, saying a gratitude prayer before bed, or simply taking a few deep breaths and silently expressing gratitude. Find a practice that resonates with you and make it a regular part of your routine.

The Power of Self-Reflection

Self-reflection is the process of introspection and examining one's thoughts, feelings, and actions. It is a valuable tool for personal growth and self-improvement. As a working woman, self-reflection can help you gain clarity, identify areas for growth, and make conscious choices that align with your values and goals.

Self-reflection allows you to pause and evaluate your experiences, both positive and negative. It helps you understand your strengths and weaknesses, enabling you to make informed decisions and take actions that will lead to personal and professional success. By regularly engaging in self-reflection, you can become more self-aware, develop a deeper understanding of yourself, and make intentional choices that support your well-being and happiness.

Ways to Practice Self-Reflection

Here are some strategies to incorporate self-reflection into your routine:

1. **Journaling**: Set aside dedicated time each day or week to journal about your thoughts, feelings, and experiences. Use this time to reflect on your achievements, challenges, and lessons learned. Writing can help you gain clarity and perspective, allowing you to make more informed decisions and take purposeful actions.

2. **Meditation and Mindfulness**: Incorporate mindfulness and meditation practices into your daily routine. These practices can help you cultivate a sense of presence and awareness, allowing you to observe your thoughts and emotions without judgment. By creating space for stillness and reflection, you can gain valuable insights into yourself and your experiences.

3. **Seek Feedback**: Actively seek feedback from trusted colleagues, mentors, or friends. Their perspectives can provide valuable insights into your strengths and areas for improvement. Be open to constructive criticism and use it as an opportunity for growth and self-reflection.

4. **Set Goals and Evaluate Progress**: Regularly set goals for yourself and evaluate your progress. Take the time to reflect on your achievements, setbacks, and lessons learned. This practice will help you stay focused, motivated, and aligned with your long-term aspirations.

The Power of Gratitude and Self-Reflection Combined

Practicing gratitude and self-reflection together can be a powerful combination. When you express gratitude, you acknowledge the positive aspects of your life, fostering a sense of contentment and appreciation. Self-reflection, on the other hand, allows you to gain insights into your thoughts, emotions, and actions, leading to personal growth and self-improvement.

By combining these practices, you can develop a deeper understanding of yourself and your experiences. You can cultivate a positive mindset, appreciate the present moment, and make conscious choices that align with your values and goals. This combination can help you navigate the challenges of balancing work and fitness, maintain a healthy work-life integration, and ultimately lead a fulfilling and empowered life as a working woman.

Remember, practicing gratitude and self-reflection is a journey, and it takes time and commitment. Start small, be consistent, and be gentle with yourself. Over time, you will reap the benefits of these practices and experience a positive transformation in your life.

Empowering Your Journey

12.1 Embracing Your Strength and Power

As a working woman, you have already proven your strength and power by successfully balancing your career and fitness journey. In this final section of the book, we will explore how you can continue to embrace your strength and power, set new goals, challenge yourself, and inspire and support others along the way.

Embracing Your Strength

Throughout this book, you have learned about the physical and mental benefits of exercise, the importance of self-care, and the strategies for balancing work and fitness. Now is the time to truly embrace your strength and acknowledge the progress you have made. Take a moment to reflect on how far you have come and the obstacles you have overcome. Celebrate your achievements, no matter how big or small they may seem.

Embracing your strength also means recognizing your worth and value as a woman in the workplace. You have unique skills, talents, and perspectives that contribute to the success of your team and organization. Believe in yourself and the power you possess to make a difference in your career and in the lives of others.

Setting New Goals

With your newfound strength and power, it's important to continue setting new goals for yourself. Goals provide direction and motivation, and they keep you focused on your journey. Reflect on what you have already accomplished and think about what you want to achieve next.

When setting new goals, make sure they are specific, measurable, attainable, relevant, and time-bound (SMART). For example, instead of saying, "I want to get stronger," set a goal like, "I want to increase my deadlift by 10 pounds within the next three months." This way, you have a clear target to work towards and can track your progress along the way.

Remember to challenge yourself with your goals. Pushing beyond your comfort zone is where growth happens. Whether it's aiming for a promotion at work, completing a challenging fitness event, or learning a new skill, set goals that inspire and motivate you to become the best version of yourself.

Challenging Yourself

As you continue on your fitness journey, it's important to challenge yourself regularly. This means stepping out of your comfort zone and trying new things. It could be experimenting with different workout styles, taking on new responsibilities at work, or seeking opportunities for personal and professional growth.

Challenging yourself not only keeps things exciting and prevents boredom, but it also helps you discover new strengths and capabilities. Don't be afraid to take risks and embrace the unknown. Remember, growth happens outside of your comfort zone.

Inspiring and Supporting Others

As a strong and powerful woman, you have the ability to inspire and support others on their own fitness and career journeys. Share your experiences, successes, and challenges with those around you. Be a role model and show others what is possible when you prioritize your health and well-being.

Supporting others can be as simple as offering words of encouragement, sharing resources and knowledge, or being a listening ear. Lift others up and celebrate their achievements. By creating a supportive community, you not only help others succeed but also create a network of like-minded individuals who can inspire and motivate you in return.

Continuing Your Fitness Journey

Your fitness journey is not a destination but a lifelong commitment to your health and well-being. As you embrace your strength and power, set new goals, challenge yourself, and inspire others, remember to continue evolving and growing.

Stay curious and open-minded. Keep learning about new fitness trends, techniques, and research. Adapt your routines and strategies as needed to ensure continued progress. Surround yourself with positive influences and seek out opportunities for personal and professional development.

Most importantly, remember that your fitness journey is unique to you. Embrace your individuality and listen to your body. Trust yourself and the power you possess to create a fulfilling and balanced life.

Congratulations on completing "The Power Hustle: A Guide to Balancing Work and Fitness for Women." You are now equipped with the knowledge, tools, and mindset to thrive in both your career and fitness journey. Embrace your strength and power, set new goals, challenge yourself, inspire and support others, and continue your fitness journey with confidence and determination. You have the power to create the life you desire.

12.2 Setting New Goals and Challenging Yourself

Setting goals is an essential part of any fitness journey. It gives you something to strive for and helps you stay motivated and focused. As a working woman, it's important to set new goals and challenge yourself regularly to continue progressing and growing in your fitness journey. In this section, we will explore the importance of setting new goals, how to set them effectively, and strategies to challenge yourself along the way.

The Importance of Setting New Goals

Setting new goals is crucial for several reasons. Firstly, it helps you maintain your motivation and enthusiasm for exercise. When you achieve a goal, it's natural to feel a sense of accomplishment and satisfaction. However, once that goal is reached, it's important to set new ones to keep the momentum going.

Secondly, setting new goals allows you to continue pushing yourself and making progress. Without new goals, it's easy to fall into a comfort zone and plateau in your fitness journey. By setting new challenges, you can continue to improve your strength, endurance, and overall fitness level.

Lastly, setting new goals helps you stay focused and committed. When you have a clear target in mind, it becomes easier to prioritize your workouts and make time for exercise. It also provides a sense of direction and purpose, making it less likely for you to get sidetracked or lose sight of your fitness goals.

How to Set Goals Effectively

To set goals effectively, it's important to follow the SMART goal-setting framework:

1. **Specific**: Your goals should be clear and well-defined. Instead of saying, "I want to get stronger," specify what you want to achieve, such as "I want to increase my squat weight by 10 pounds."

2. **Measurable**: Your goals should be quantifiable so that you can track your progress. For example, instead of saying, "I want to run faster," set a specific time goal, such as "I want to complete a 5K race in under 30 minutes."

3. **Achievable**: Your goals should be realistic and attainable. While it's important to challenge yourself, setting unrealistic goals can lead to frustration and disappointment. Consider your current fitness level and set goals that are challenging but within reach.

4. **Relevant**: Your goals should align with your overall fitness journey and personal aspirations. Make sure your goals are meaningful to you and will contribute to your overall well-being and happiness.

5. **Time-bound**: Your goals should have a specific timeframe for completion. Setting a deadline creates a sense of urgency and helps you stay focused. For example, instead of saying, "I want to do a pull-up," set a timeframe, such as "I want to do a pull-up within three months."

By following the SMART framework, you can set goals that are clear, measurable, achievable, relevant, and time-bound, increasing your chances of success.

Strategies to Challenge Yourself

Once you have set your goals, it's important to challenge yourself along the way to keep progressing. Here are some strategies to help you do that:

1. **Progressive Overload**: Gradually increase the intensity, duration, or frequency of your workouts. This could mean adding more weight to your strength training exercises, increasing the distance or speed of your runs, or adding an extra day of exercise to your weekly routine. By consistently challenging your body, you will continue to see improvements.

2. **Try New Workouts**: Incorporate different types of workouts into your routine to challenge your body in new ways. If you primarily do cardio exercises, try adding strength training or yoga sessions to your schedule. Experimenting with different workouts not only keeps things interesting but also helps you work different muscle groups and improve overall fitness.

3. **Set Performance-Based Goals**: Instead of solely focusing on aesthetic goals, such as weight loss or body measurements, set goals that are performance-based. For example, aim to complete a certain number of push-ups or run a specific distance within a given time. Performance-based goals shift the focus from appearance to what your body can do, which can be incredibly empowering.

4. **Join Challenges or Competitions**: Participating in fitness challenges or competitions can provide an extra level of motivation and accountability. Whether it's a virtual race, a step challenge with friends, or a local fitness competition, these events can push you to work harder and achieve new milestones.

5. **Track Your Progress**: Keep a record of your workouts, measurements, and achievements. Tracking your progress allows you to see how far you've come and provides a visual reminder of your accomplishments. It can also help you identify areas where you may need to adjust your approach or set new goals.

Remember, challenging yourself doesn't mean pushing yourself to the point of exhaustion or injury. It's about finding the right balance between pushing your limits and listening to your body. Be mindful of your body's signals and make adjustments as needed.

By setting new goals and challenging yourself regularly, you can continue to grow and evolve in your fitness journey. Embrace the power of setting new goals, and let them inspire you to reach new heights in both your work and fitness life.

12.3 Inspiring and Supporting Others

As a working woman who has successfully balanced work and fitness, you have the power to inspire and support others on their own fitness journeys. By sharing your experiences, knowledge, and encouragement, you can help empower other women to prioritize their health and well-being. In this section, we will explore various ways in which you can inspire and support others in their pursuit of a balanced and healthy lifestyle.

Lead by Example

One of the most effective ways to inspire others is by leading by example. When people see you consistently making time for exercise and prioritizing your health, they are more likely to be motivated to do the same. Be a role model for those around you by demonstrating the positive impact that fitness has on your life. Share your success stories, both big and small, and let others see the joy and fulfillment that comes from taking care of yourself.

Share Your Knowledge

Another way to inspire and support others is by sharing your knowledge and expertise. Offer guidance and advice to those who are just starting their fitness journey or struggling to find the right balance. Share tips on time management, goal setting, and creating effective exercise routines. Educate others about the benefits of exercise and the importance of self-care. By sharing your knowledge, you can empower others to make informed decisions about their health and fitness.

Be a Supportive Listener

Sometimes, all someone needs is a listening ear and a supportive voice. Be there for others when they need to talk about their challenges, frustrations, or successes. Show empathy and understanding, and offer words of encouragement and motivation. Let them know that they are not alone in their struggles and that you believe in their ability to overcome obstacles. By being a supportive listener, you can provide the emotional support that others may need to stay motivated and committed to their fitness goals.

Create a Supportive Community

Building a supportive community is essential for long-term success in balancing work and fitness. Encourage others to join you in your fitness endeavors and create a network of like-minded individuals who can support and motivate each other. This can be done through fitness classes, workout groups, or online communities. By fostering a sense of belonging and camaraderie, you can create an environment where everyone feels supported and inspired to achieve their fitness goals.

Celebrate Milestones and Achievements

When someone achieves a milestone or reaches a goal, celebrate their success! Acknowledge their hard work and dedication, and let them know how proud you are of their accomplishments. This can be done through small gestures like sending a congratulatory message or organizing a group celebration. By celebrating milestones and achievements, you not only show support for others but also inspire them to continue pushing themselves and striving for more.

Offer Accountability

Accountability is crucial when it comes to maintaining consistency in fitness routines. Offer to be an accountability partner for someone who is struggling to stay on track. Check in with them regularly, offer words of encouragement, and hold them accountable for their commitments. This can be done through regular check-ins, shared workout sessions, or even setting joint fitness goals. By providing accountability, you can help others stay motivated and committed to their fitness journey.

Volunteer and Give Back

Inspiring and supporting others can extend beyond your immediate circle. Consider volunteering your time and expertise to organizations or initiatives that promote health and fitness. This could involve leading fitness classes, mentoring others, or participating in community events. By giving back to your community, you not only inspire others but also contribute to the overall well-being of those around you.

Be Patient and Understanding

Lastly, it is important to be patient and understanding when supporting others on their fitness journey. Recognize that everyone's path is unique, and progress may not always be linear. Be patient with setbacks and challenges, and offer support and guidance without judgment. Understand that change takes time and that everyone has their own pace. By being patient and understanding, you create a safe and non-judgmental space for others to grow and thrive.

Remember, inspiring and supporting others is a powerful way to make a positive impact in the lives of those around you. By sharing your experiences, knowledge, and encouragement, you can empower others to prioritize their health and well-being. Together, we can create a community of strong, empowered, and balanced women who are ready to take on any challenge that comes their way.

12.4 Continuing Your Fitness Journey

Congratulations! You have come a long way in your fitness journey. You have learned how to balance work and fitness, prioritize self-care, and overcome obstacles. Now, it's time to focus on continuing your fitness journey and making it a lifelong commitment. In this section, we will explore strategies to help you stay motivated, set new goals, and maintain your progress.

Embracing Consistency

Consistency is key when it comes to maintaining your fitness journey. It's important to make exercise a regular part of your routine, just like brushing your teeth or eating breakfast. By consistently incorporating exercise into your daily life, you will not only maintain your progress but also continue to reap the benefits of a healthy and active lifestyle.

One way to ensure consistency is by scheduling your workouts in advance. Treat your exercise sessions as important appointments that cannot be missed. Set specific days and times for your workouts and stick to them as much as possible. By making exercise a non-negotiable part of your schedule, you are more likely to follow through and stay committed.

Setting New Goals

As you continue your fitness journey, it's important to set new goals to keep yourself motivated and challenged. Goals give you something to strive for and help you measure your progress. When setting new goals, make sure they are realistic, specific, and measurable.

Consider setting both short-term and long-term goals. Short-term goals can be achieved within a few weeks or months, while long-term goals may take several months or even years to accomplish. Short-term goals can help you stay motivated and provide a sense of accomplishment along the way, while long-term goals give you something to work towards in the future.

When setting goals, focus on different aspects of fitness. For example, you may set a strength-related goal, such as increasing the amount of weight you can lift or the number of push-ups you can do. You could also set a cardiovascular goal, such as running a certain distance or improving your time in a specific exercise. By diversifying your goals, you can continue to challenge yourself and improve in various areas of fitness.

Trying New Activities

To keep your fitness journey exciting and prevent boredom, consider trying new activities or workouts. Exploring different types of exercise not only keeps things interesting but also challenges your body in new ways.

There are countless options to choose from, depending on your interests and preferences. You could try a new fitness class, such as kickboxing, dance, or yoga. If you enjoy outdoor activities, consider hiking, cycling, or swimming. You could also experiment with different workout formats, such as circuit training, HIIT (high-intensity interval training), or Pilates.

By trying new activities, you may discover a new passion or find a workout that you truly enjoy. This can make your fitness journey more enjoyable and sustainable in the long run.

Seeking Support and Accountability

Maintaining your fitness journey becomes easier when you have a support system in place. Surround yourself with like-minded individuals who share your commitment to health and fitness. This could be friends, family members, or even online communities. Having people who understand and support your goals can provide motivation and encouragement when you need it most.

In addition to support, accountability can also play a crucial role in staying on track. Consider finding an accountability partner or joining a fitness group where you can share your progress, challenges, and successes. Knowing that others are counting on you can help you stay committed and motivated.

Reflecting and Celebrating

Take time to reflect on your fitness journey and celebrate your achievements. Look back at how far you have come and acknowledge the hard work and dedication you have put into your health and well-being. Celebrate your milestones, whether it's reaching a weight loss goal, completing a challenging workout, or improving your overall fitness level.

Celebrating your achievements not only boosts your confidence but also reinforces the positive habits you have developed. It reminds you of the progress you have made and motivates you to continue pushing forward.

Embracing a Growth Mindset

Finally, as you continue your fitness journey, it's important to embrace a growth mindset. Understand that setbacks and plateaus are a normal part of any journey. Instead of getting discouraged, view them as opportunities for growth and learning.

When faced with challenges, remind yourself of the progress you have already made and the obstacles you have overcome. Use setbacks as motivation to push harder and find new ways to overcome obstacles. Remember that every step forward, no matter how small, is a step in the right direction.

By embracing a growth mindset, you will continue to evolve and improve on your fitness journey. You will be open to new possibilities and challenges, and you will continue to grow stronger, both physically and mentally.

Congratulations on reaching this point in your fitness journey! Remember, it's not just about reaching a destination but about embracing the process and making fitness a lifelong commitment. By continuing to prioritize your health and well-being, you are empowering yourself to live a balanced and fulfilling life. Keep up the great work!